Copyright © 2022 Matthew Thrush

Total Gut Makeover: Crohn's Disease: 125 Recipes & Foods Proven To Be Neutral Or Beneficial For Relieving Crohn's Disease | 21-Day Meal Plan Included With Alternative Medicine For Faster Recovery

All rights reserved. No part of this guide may be reproduced in any form without permission in writing from the publisher except in the case of brief quotations embodied in critical articles or reviews.

King of Kings Publishing
20212 Champion Forest Dr. #303
Spring, TX 77379
www.kingofkingspublishing.com
@kingofkingspublishing

Legal & Disclaimer
The information contained in this book and its contents is not designed to replace or take the place of any form of medical or professional advice; and is not meant to replace the need for independent medical, financial, legal or other professional advice or services, as may be required.

The content and information in this book has been provided for educational and entertainment purposes only. The content and information contained in this book has been compiled from sources deemed reliable, and it is accurate to the best of the Author's knowledge, information and belief. However, the Author cannot guarantee its accuracy and validity and cannot be held liable for any errors and/or omissions. Further, changes are periodically made to this book as and when needed. Where appropriate and/or necessary, you must consult a professional (including but not limited to your doctor, attorney, financial advisor or such other professional advisor) before using any of the suggested remedies, techniques, or information in this book.

Upon using the contents and information contained in this book, you agree to hold harmless the Author from and against any damages, costs, and expenses, including any legal fees potentially resulting from the application of any of the information provided by this book. This disclaimer applies to any loss, damages or injury caused by the use and application, whether directly or indirectly, of any advice or information presented, whether for breach of contract, tort, negligence, personal injury, criminal intent, or under any other cause of action.

You agree to accept all risks of using the information presented inside this book.

You agree that by continuing to read this book, where appropriate and/or necessary, you shall consult a professional (including but not limited to your doctor, attorney, or financial advisor or such other advisor as needed) before using any of the suggested remedies, techniques, or information in this book.

TABLE OF CONTENTS

Introduction I

CHAPTER TWO: Snacks 1
Roasted Chickpeas 2
Fruit and Nut Bars 3
Cucumber Avocado Tea Sandwiches 4
Chocolate Hummus 5
Sweet Potato Chips 6
Parmesan Garlic Kale Chips 7
Spicy Roasted Edamame 8
Trail Mix 9
Banana Sushi 10
Apple Nachos 11
Cucumber Bites 12
Cherry Tomatoes with Basil 13
Carrot Sticks with Hummus 14
Celery Sticks with Peanut Butter 15
Cauliflower Popcorn 16
Edamame 17
Fruit Kabobs 18
Grapefruit with Honey 19
Cantaloupe with Cottage Cheese 20
Orange with Almond Butter 21
Peach with Yogurt 22
Pineapple with Coconut Milk 23
Strawberry with Balsamic Vinegar 24
Watermelon with Mint 25
Veggie Chips 26

CHAPTER THREE: Breakfast 27
Banana Bread Overnight Oats 28
Blueberry Almond Pancakes 29
Breakfast Tacos 30
Cinnamon Roll Baked Oatmeal 31
Peach and Arugula Salad 32
Banana Oatmeal 33
Blueberry Muffins 34

TABLE OF CONTENTS

Chocolate Chip Pancakes..35
Cinnamon Rolls...36
Egg Breakfast Sandwich..37
Fruit Salad...38
Green Smoothie..39
Grilled Cheese Sandwich..40
Quiche...41
Tomato Soup...42
Omelet with Vegetables.. 43
Scrambled Eggs with Spinach and Cheese..44
Sausage and Egg Breakfast Burrito..45
Banana Pancakes...46
Quinoa Breakfast Bowl..47
Breakfast Smoothie...48
Greek Yogurt with Fruit and Honey...49
Avocado Toast...50
Smoked Salmon Bagel..51
Yogurt Parfait...52

CHAPTER FOUR: Lunch...53
Quinoa Veggie Bowl..54
Spicy Thai Peanut Noodles...55
Greek Yogurt Chicken Salad...56
Spicy Black Bean Soup...57
Curried Lentil Soup..58
Tomato Basil Soup 59
White Bean Chicken Chili..60
Spicy Black Bean Burger with Avocado Mayo and Roasted Sweet Potato Wedges...........61
Quinoa Salad with Roasted Vegetables 62
Sautéed Shrimp with Zucchini Noodles and Pesto...63
Thai Chicken Wraps..64
Turkey and Apple Sandwich on Gluten-Free Bread..65
Spaghetti Squash with Tomato Sauce..66
Eggplant Parmesan...67

TABLE OF CONTENTS

Turkey Wrap..68
Quinoa Pilaf..69
Chickpea Salad...70
Garlic Mashed Potatoes..71
Meat and Vegetable Rollups...72
Garden Veggie Soup...73
Quinoa Salad with Cranberries and Feta..74
Potato Soup with Bacon, Cheese, and Scallions..75
Pink Salmon Salad with Vegetables..76
Spicy Sausage and Kale Soup..77
Tomato Basil Chicken..78

CHAPTER FIVE: Dinner..79
Chicken and Broccoli Stir Fry..80
Grilled Chicken with Roasted Vegetables...81
Crockpot Honey Garlic Chicken..82
One Pot BBQ Chicken and Quinoa...83
Salmon with Roasted Brussels Sprouts..84
Beef Stir Fry with Broccoli and Brown Rice...85
Turkey Burger with Sweet Potato Fries...86
Quinoa Salad with Grilled Chicken..88
Lentil Soup..90
Spaghetti Squash with Turkey Meat Sauce..91
Roasted Chicken with Roasted Vegetables..92
Salmon with Quinoa and Roasted Vegetables..93
Chicken Curry with Coconut Milk and Rice...94
Beef Stew with Potatoes and Carrots..95
Turkey Chili...96
Baked Ham With Sweet Potato Casserole and Green Beans......................97
Shepherd's Pie..99
Salmon Cakes with Roasted Vegetables..100
Beef Stroganoff...101
Meatloaf with Mashed Potatoes and Carrots..102
Roasted Turkey Breast with Stuffing and Green Beans..............................103
Roasted Pork Loin with Sweet Potatoes and Apples..................................105
Vegetable Lasagna...106
Beef Stew..107
Chicken Pot Pie...108

TABLE OF CONTENTS

CHAPTER SIX: Desserts...109
Chocolate Chip Banana Bread...110
Blueberry Crisp..111
Brownies..112
Chocolate Chip Cookies..113
Oatmeal Chocolate Chip Cookies...114
Peanut Butter Cookies...115
Sugar Cookies..116
Oreo Cheesecake Bites..117
Strawberry Shortcake..118
Chocolate Covered Strawberries..119
Peach Cobbler..120
Vanilla Pudding..122
Crème Brulee...123
Tiramisu...124
Flan...125
Scones...126
Frozen Fruit Sorbet...127
Chocolate Mousse..128
Strawberry Cheesecake Bites..129
Lemon Meringue Smoothie..130
Frozen Yogurt Bites..131
Angel Pecan Pie...132
Chocolate Pudding...133
Blueberry Cobbler...134
Peach Crisp..135

TABLE OF CONTENTS

21-Day Meal Plan..136

Day 1:..137
   Snack: Fruit and Nut Bars.. 3
   Breakfast: Banana Oatmeal..33
   Lunch: Tomato Basil Soup..59
   Dinner: Beef Stir Fry with Broccoli and Brown Rice................................85
   Dessert: Sugar Cookies...116

Day 2:..137
   Snack: Banana Sushi..10
   Breakfast: Quinoa Breakfast Bowl..47
   Lunch: Curried Lentil Soup...58
   Dinner: Turkey Chili..97
   Dessert: Lemon Meringue Smoothie...130

Day 3:..137
   Snack: Apple Nachos..11
   Breakfast: Breakfast Tacos...30
   Lunch: Spicy Thai Peanut Noodles...55
   Dinner: Shepherd's Pie...99
   Dessert: Brownies...112

Day 4:..137
   Snack: Edamame..17
   Breakfast: Banana Pancakes..46
   Lunch: Quinoa Pilaf..69
   Dinner: Baked Ham with Sweet Potato Casserole and Green Beans............98
   Dessert: Oreo Cheesecake Bites...117

Day 5:..138
   Snack: Watermelon with Mint..25
   Breakfast: Blueberry Almond Pancakes...29
   Lunch: White Bean Chicken Chili..60
   Dinner: Meatloaf with Mashed Potatoes and Carrots...........................102
   Dessert: Tiramisu..124

TABLE OF CONTENTS

21-Day Meal Plan..136

Day 6:..138
  Snack: Orange with Almond Butter..21
  Breakfast: Omelet with Vegetables..43
  Lunch: Thai Chicken Wraps..64
  Dinner: Spaghetti Squash with Turkey Meat Sauce..92
  Dessert: Peach Cobbler..120..120

Day 7:..138
  Snack: Cauliflower..16
  Breakfast: Green Smoothie..39
  Lunch: Eggplant Parmesan..67
  Dinner: Salmon Cakes with Roasted Vegetables..100
  Dessert: Angel Pecan Pie..132

Day 8:..138
  Snack: Veggie Chips..26
  Breakfast: Peach and Arugula Salad..32
  Lunch: Turkey and Apple Sandwich on Gluten-Free Bread..65
  Dinner: Chicken Pot Pie..108
  Dessert: Flan..125

Day 9:..138
  Snack: Celery Sticks with Peanut Butter..15
  Breakfast: Quiche..41
  Lunch: Spicy Black Bean Soup..57
  Dinner: Turkey Burger with Sweet Potato Fries..86
  Dessert: Strawberry Shortcake..118

Day 10:..139
  Snack: Roasted Chickpeas..2
  Breakfast: Scrambled Eggs with Spinach and Cheese..44
  Lunch: Sautéed Shrimp with Zucchini Noodles and Pesto..63
  Dinner: Chicken and Broccoli Stir Fry..80
  Dessert: Blueberry Crisp..111

TABLE OF CONTENTS

21-Day Meal Plan..136

Day 11:..139
   Snack: Cantaloupe with Cottage Cheese.................................20
   Breakfast: Grilled Cheese Sandwich...40
   Lunch: Meat and Vegetable Rollups..72
   Dinner: One Pot BBQ Chicken and Quinoa..............................83
   Dessert: Chocolate Mousse...129

Day 12:..139
   Snack: Parmesan Garlic Kale Chips..7
   Breakfast: Cinnamon Roll Baked Oatmeal...............................31
   Lunch: Pink Salmon Salad with Vegetables.............................76
   Dinner: Salmon with Quinoa and Roasted Vegetables...........94
   Dessert: Chocolate Chip Cookies..113

Day 13:..139
   Snack: Cucumber Bites...12
   Breakfast: Egg Breakfast Sandwich..37
   Lunch: Spicy Black Bean Burger with Avocado Mayo
      and Roasted Sweet Potato Wedges....................................61
   Dinner: Crockpot Honey Garlic Chicken..................................82
   Dessert: Peanut Butter Cookies..115

Day 14:..140
   Snack: Cucumber Avocado Tea Sandwiches.............................4
   Breakfast: Sausage and Egg Breakfast Burrito.......................45
   Lunch: Quinoa Salad with Roasted Vegetables......................62
   Dinner: Grilled Chicken with Roasted Vegetables..................81
   Dessert: Scones...126

TABLE OF CONTENTS

21-Day Meal Plan..136

Day 15:..140
   Snack: Trail Mix... 9
   Breakfast: Banana Bread Overnight Oats.......................................28
   Lunch: Spaghetti Squash with Tomato Sauce................................66
   Dinner: Lentil Soup...91
   Dessert: Peach Crisp...135

Day 16:..140
   Snack: Carrot Sticks with Hummus..14
   Breakfast: Avocado Toast...50
   Lunch: Greek Yogurt Chicken Salad..56
   Dinner: Roasted Pork Loin with Sweet Potatoes and Apples.......105
   Dessert: Chocolate Chip Banana Bread..110

Day 17:..140
   Snack: Cherry Tomatoes with Basil..13
   Breakfast: Blueberry Muffins..34
   Lunch: Turkey Wrap...68
   Dinner: Quinoa Salad with Grilled Chicken...................................89
   Dessert: Vanilla Pudding..122

Day 18:..141
   Snack: Sweet Potato Chips... 6
   Breakfast: Cinnamon Rolls..36
   Lunch: Chickpea Salad..70
   Dinner: Roasted Chicken with Roasted Vegetables......................93
   Dessert: Chocolate Covered Strawberries...................................119

Day 19:..141
   Snack: Fruit Kabobs...18
   Breakfast: Chocolate Chip Pancakes..35
   Lunch: Tomato Basil Chicken..78
   Dinner: Beef Stew with Potatoes and Carrots...............................96
   Dessert: Frozen Yogurt Bites...131

TABLE OF CONTENTS

21-Day Meal Plan..136

Day 20:..141
    Snack: Pineapple with Coconut Milk..23
    Breakfast: Banana Pancakes...46
    Lunch: Garlic Mashed Potatoes..71
    Dinner: Beef Stroganoff...101
    Dessert: Crème Brulee...123

Day 21:..141
    Snack: Strawberry with Balsamic Vinegar.......................................24
    Breakfast: Quinoa Breakfast Bowl..47
    Lunch: Quinoa Salad with Cranberries and Feta.............................74
    Dinner: Roasted Turkey Breast with Stuffing and Green Beans....103
    Dessert: Blueberry Cobbler...134

About the Author..142

Rapid healing made easy...143

Operation Love..147

About Matthew Thrush..148

Also by Matthew Thrush..150

Index...152

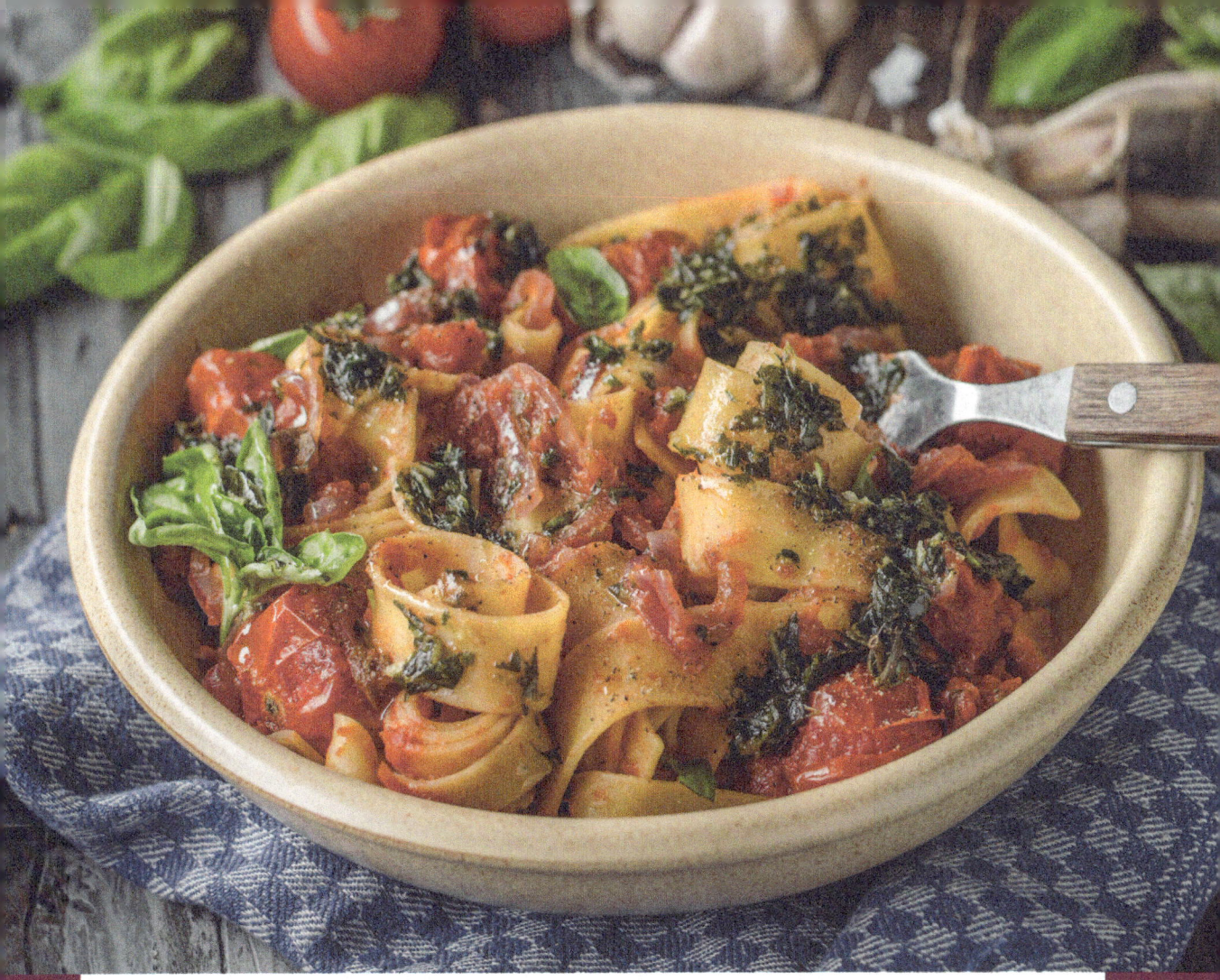

CHAPTER ONE: INTRODUCTION

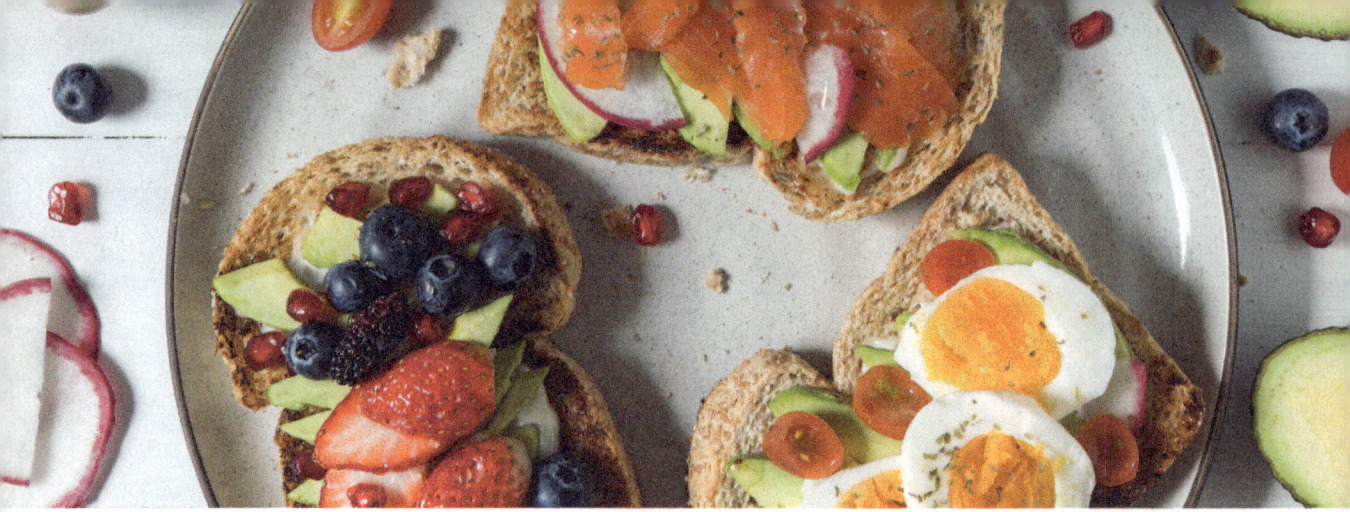

INTRODUCTION

So here you are, holding this book in your hands because chances are that you or a loved one has been diagnosed with Crohn's disease. If you're feeling overwhelmed about what to do now, then rest easy because you're in the right place. This book is here to help!

You are definitely not alone with your diagnosis. Over 780,000 Americans have Crohn's disease, with about 1 in 10,000 people getting newly diagnosed every single year. And even though you might not have given Crohn's much thought until your tummy started acting up, your head is probably now reeling with a million questions about how you've gotten here and what to do about it. Questions like how you are going to live with this, and what to do to ease your discomfort, are at the very top of the list.

But first, let's dive into this question: what is Crohn's disease?

As frustrating as it is, Crohn's is a chronic condition for which there is no cure. It's an inflammatory disease of the intestines that causes ulcerations of the small and large intestines. "Ouch" is right! It's also closely related to another chronic condition called ulcerative colitis, which together are referred to as inflammatory bowel disease.

The bad news is that there is no known medical cure, but the good news is that you haven't been sentenced to live in constant pain. Crohn's disease fluctuates between remission and relapse, and remission is where we want to be!

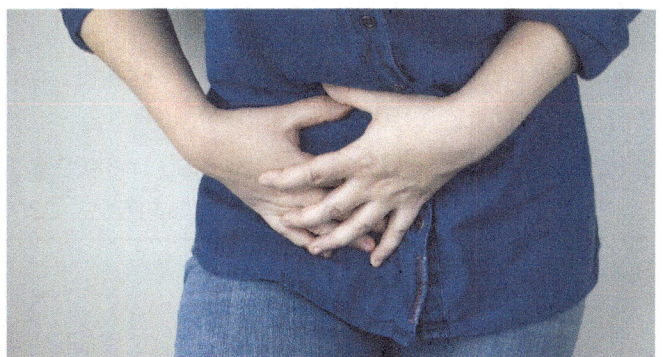

WHY ME?

How did you get it? Well, medical experts don't have a cut-and-dried answer for you on that one. Perhaps it was a genetic luck of the draw, or a hefty pile of risk factors at play. Some scientists believe that the infection is caused by certain strains of bacteria, but the disease is not contagious. Although diet can affect symptoms of the disease, it's not responsible for causing Crohn's.

Men and women are equally affected by inflammatory bowel disease, and Crohn's tends to be more common in relatives of patients with Crohn's disease. In fact, if you have a relative who has the disease, your risk of developing Crohn's is at least ten times higher than that of the general population.

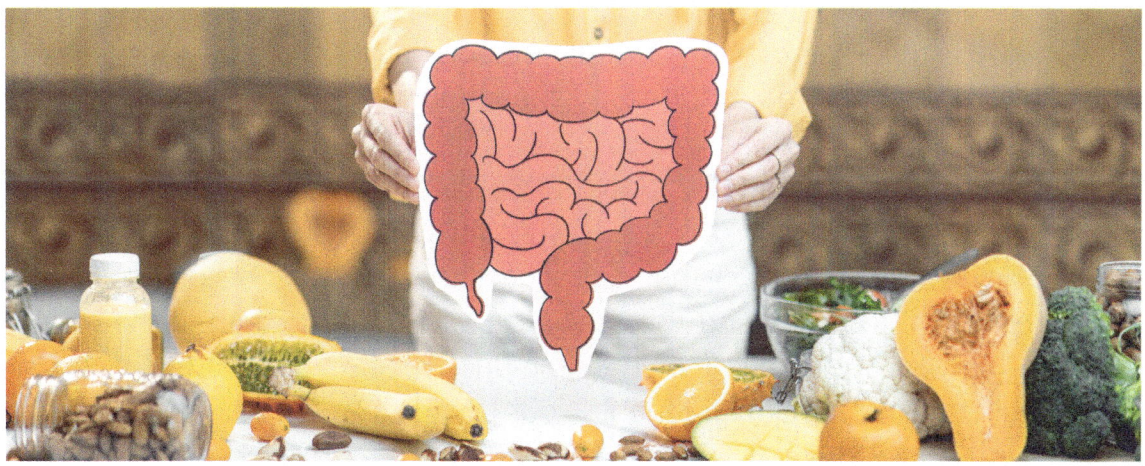

Risk factors can play a part, too. Although Crohn's can occur at any time, it develops for most people while they are under the age of thirty. And although it can affect any ethnic group, whites have the highest risk, especially amongst people of Jewish descent. Smoking makes a solid appearance on the risk factors for Crohn's, though it is one of the most controllable risk factors for developing the condition.

If you smoke, think twice about stopping now, because it also leads to a much higher risk of having a severe form of the disease. While nonsteroidal anti-inflammatory medications don't cause Crohn's disease, they can lead to inflammation of the bowel, which will make Crohn's worse.

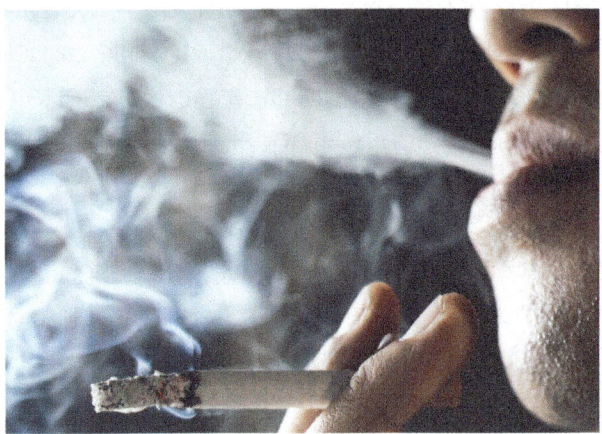
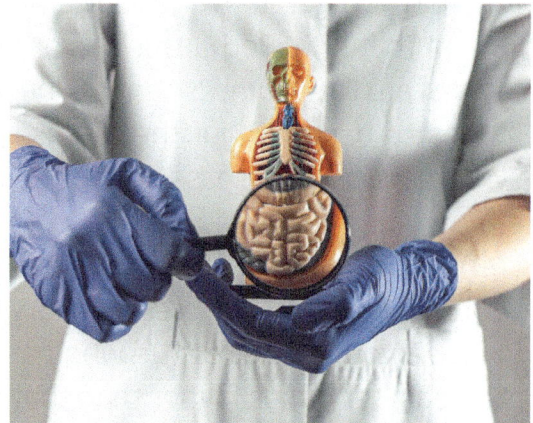

The one thing that is certain is that your intestinal immune system isn't falling in line. With inflammatory bowel diseases, the immune system in the intestines is abnormally and chronically activated.

Usually, the body's healthy immune system is activated in order to fend off harmful invaders, causing inflammation where the activation occurs to fight off the foreign threat and defend the body. But with Crohn's, there is no foreign invader, just an overreaction of the immune system that leads to chronic inflammation and ulceration. Suddenly, your body is a little confused about who the bad guy is!

LET'S TALK SYMPTOMS

Your overall goal is to be symptom-free, right? That's what we're aiming for here—long periods of remission in which you don't have to suffer the negative consequences of Crohn's disease because they're definitely no fun. Everyone's body is different, and the symptoms of Crohn's will depend on its location, extent of spread, and severity of the inflammation.

Abdominal pain: Your abdomen is the core of your body. No one wants to be hindered by abdominal pain. Being doubled over at work, or uncomfortable when eating—nothing puts a damper on being productive or trying to enjoy yourself more than a cramped-up gut.

Diarrhea: The dreaded symptom that people shy away from talking about, and with good reason! Discussing a burning bottom or a mad dash to the bathroom doesn't exactly make for easy conversation. And to make matters worse, diarrhea can exacerbate other symptoms like cramping and dehydration.

Weight loss: This isn't the good kind of slimming down as a result of motivating workouts and careful diet choices. Weight loss with Crohn's comes from your digestive system not cooperating as it should.

Less common symptoms, such as poor appetite, fever, night sweats, and rectal pain, can also rear up and really make you feel like kicking Crohn's to the curb.

But fear not! Because help is on the way!

The longer you let Crohn's hang around without addressing it, the worse it will get. And since you're here reading this book, you've already taken the first step to managing your condition and living a life that isn't defined by discomfort. So, let's get you all caught up on what exactly it is that Crohn's is doing in your body and how to keep it from taking charge.

WHAT THE HECK IS GOING ON DOWN THERE?

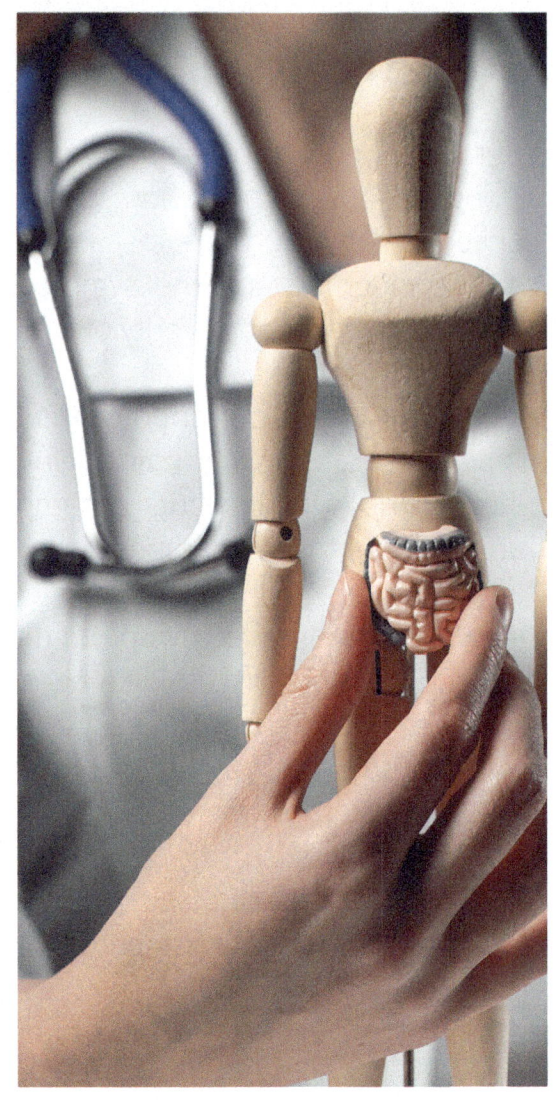

Crohn's and ulcerative colitis may both cause inflammation, but Crohn's is a heavyweight as far as affecting more areas of the body. Unlike colitis, Crohn's goes deeper than the superficial inner layers of the bowel. It can be responsible for some pretty nasty deep ulcers tucked between normal lining.

If that wasn't troublesome enough, as the disease progresses, the bowel can become increasingly narrow, which can lead to obstruction.

If the intestines become obstructed by poorly digestible food, the symptoms can continue to pile on, adding more severe abdominal cramping, nausea, vomiting, and even abdominal distention.

Deep ulcers can cause perforations in the walls of the small intestine and colon, which can lead to ulcer tunnels that might cause abdominal abscesses.

So, what's an otherwise healthy body to do? Thankfully, there are a lot of options at your fingertips, ranging from working with your doctor, to medications, to diet modifications.

The first step? Talk to the doc!

FIX ME NOW PLEASE

As with almost all ailments, talking to your doctor is the best place to start to ensure you are doing everything you can to get the best results.

An accurate diagnosis, combined with modern medicine and a holistic approach involving diet management and wellness support, means that you can actively control your Crohn's and bring it into remission.

Talk to your doctor and get all the facts for making educated choices to come up with a solid gameplan that you can fine-tune along the way.

So, you've got a chronic condition. So what? You've got this!

There are modern medical treatments to help ease the discomfort, and medications can definitely help. Your aim is to be symptom-free, so definitely use everything in your arsenal to help you battle Crohn's. But remember that reliance on medications can lead to complications of their own, which is why they are only a piece of the puzzle to put together.

The goal is to build a sustainable, healthy, and happy life that manages your condition in all the best ways possible.

Having the best nutrition to meet your needs helps modern medicine to do its thing while minimizing any other problems down the road. That's why a whole-body approach is best for increasing your quality of life.

Once your doctor has diagnosed your Crohn's disease—using laboratory blood tests that might show elevated white blood counts thar suggest inflammation, Barium X-rays to determine the severity of the disease, or a colonoscopy to detect ulcers—it's time to form a treatment plan.

DOWN THE MEDICATION RABBIT HOLE

Although there is no medication that can *cure* Crohn's disease, there are a few that can manage symptoms and prevent the disease from worsening.

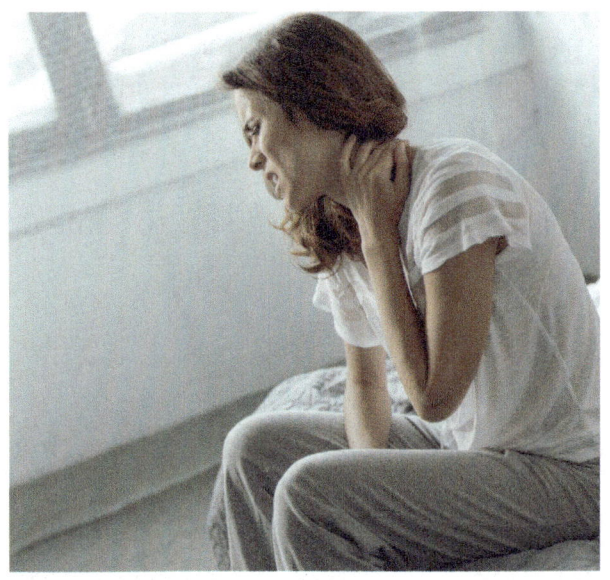

People with Crohn's will typically have flare-ups or periods of relapse in which the inflammation worsens, followed by periods of remission that last for months or even years. Remissions can occur due to treatment with medications and a healthy diet that helps manage the disease. The goal is to induce the remissions, keep them for as long as possible, and minimize any side effects any medications might cause.

Sometimes anti-inflammatory agents such as corticosteroids and 5-ASA compounds, topical antibiotics, or immunomodulators are prescribed to manage symptoms. Treatment for Crohn's has been leaning toward an early aggressive approach that aims to decrease exposure to anti-inflammatory agents and hopefully prevent any future complications.

Anti-inflammatory medications can decrease inflammation throughout the entire body, but have side effects if used for the long-term. 5-ASA is chemically similar to aspirin, and thus also an anti-inflammatory. Corticosteroids can be used to treat patients who fail to respond to 5-ASA. They are highly potent and faster acting anti-inflammatories. However, they don't appear to be helpful in prolonging remission, and they carry a slew of possible and potentially serious side effects depending on the duration of their use.

Immunomodulator medications can help control the symptoms of Crohn's but there is a risk of having weakened immunity as a result of their use.

And sometimes for severe cases, surgery can remove the diseased parts of the intestine, granting the patient possible years of being symptom-free, although inflammation frequently recurs even months or years after the surgery.

The benefits of medications carefully monitored by your doctor likely outweigh the potential risks, but there is still another thing that YOU can do to give your gut its best shot at success and ensure that you feel your very best —let's talk about food!

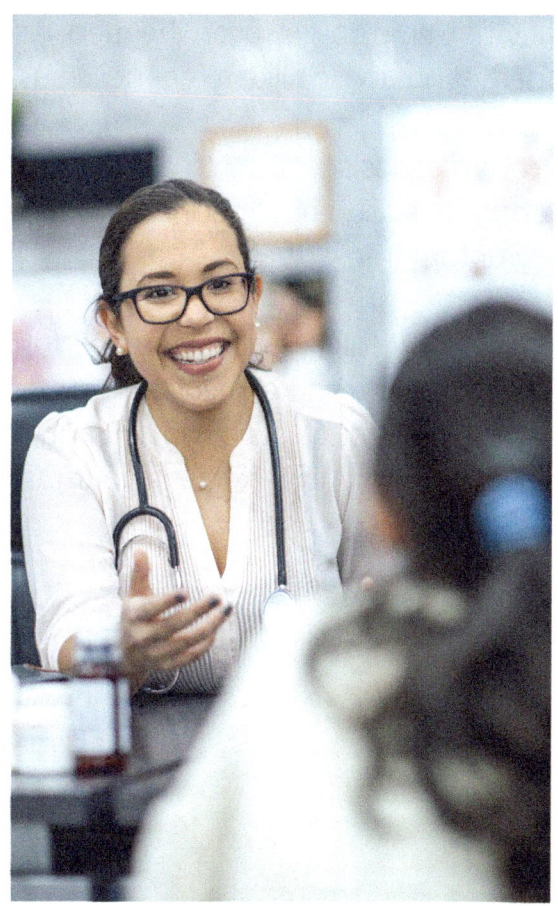

YOU ARE WHAT YOU EAT

The right foods can do a *lot* to make you feel great and keep Crohn's disease at bay. Conversely, the wrong foods can provoke those pesky symptoms into returning. That's why it's so important to eat the best foods you can to support your body.

You've been diagnosed, you now know more than you ever wanted to know about your insides, and you have a treatment plan with your doctor in place. Now it's time to help your body succeed so that you can manage your chronic condition and live your best life.

It's not time to get overwhelmed—it's time to get to work, and this is the fun part. Who doesn't like to eat delicious food that makes you feel good?

Your diagnosis is a call to action—one that is going to have you whipping up all sorts of tasty new recipes working behind the scenes to help keep you symptom-free.

Yes, you'll likely need some form of medication, some vitamins and supplements, and a regular treatment regimen with your doctor, but FOOD is where you get to have all the control. This is where you get to coax your body into remission while keeping your taste buds happy.

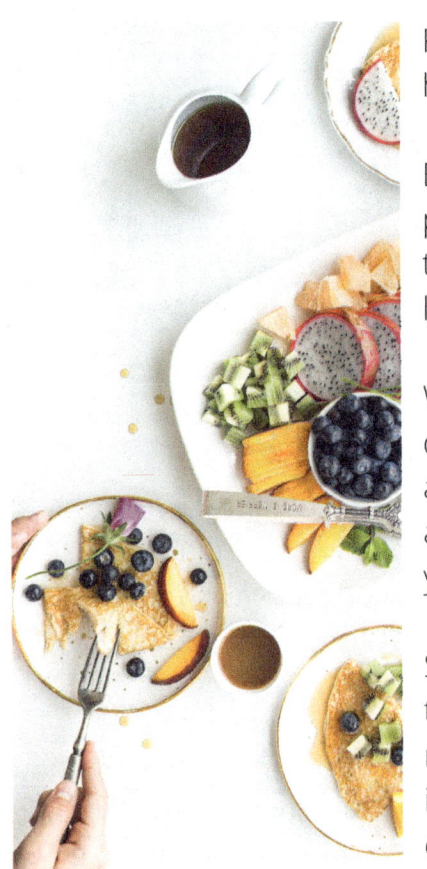

Remember, remission is the goal, but it doesn't have to be boring!

Bringing food and nutrition into your treatment plan means that you're taking a holistic approach to giving your body its best fighting chance for living a pain-free and flare-up-free life.

With the right foods and nutrients to balance your digestion, fuel your body, and steer clear of aggravating your condition, you'll be able to plan ahead and know how to lessen and even eliminate your discomfort.

Since everyone is different and no two bodies are the same, a diet plan for one person with Crohn's may not be as effective for someone else. Crohn's is a highly individualized condition, and the disease can involve different areas of the GI tract in different people.

That means that you should create your own nutritional plan based on what works for you and what doesn't.

It's helpful to keep track of your symptoms and the foods you eat so that you can see when you feel the best and when certain foods in your diet prompt or worsen symptoms.

Your focus is on reducing the recurrence of symptoms and lessening their severity, and keeping track of what works and what doesn't. All these steps can help you pinpoint a helpful strategy and not feel overwhelmed.

In general, there are a few tips to keep in mind:

Fiber: For some people suffering with Crohn's, high-fiber foods like fruits and vegetables can aggravate their GI tracts, especially since fiber is poorly digestible to begin with. If this is the case for you, then you may need to adjust your fiber intake, modifying how you consume your fiber and through which foods.

Fat: Crohn's disease can get obstruct your body's natural ability to break down and absorb fat, adding to symptomatic diarrhea and causing you more discomfort. You might be rethinking that greasy burger when it sends you running for the restroom!

Dairy: As an extra bonus, Crohn's can also make you sensitive to lactose, even if you've never had a problem with it before. If that happens to you, consuming dairy can wreak havoc on your stomach, causing abdominal cramps and diarrhea.

Water: With Crohn's already interfering with your body's ability to absorb water from your digestive tract, and potentially causing diarrhea, you are more susceptible to dehydration than a person without Crohn's. So, keep that water bottle filled and sip on it throughout the day!

But what if you aren't a five-star chef? What if you're on a budget, or don't have the time to constantly be in the kitchen? What if you can't hunt down the most elaborate ingredients, or spend your spare time earning a second degree as a nutritionist?

That's why this cookbook is staring up at you from the palms of your hands.

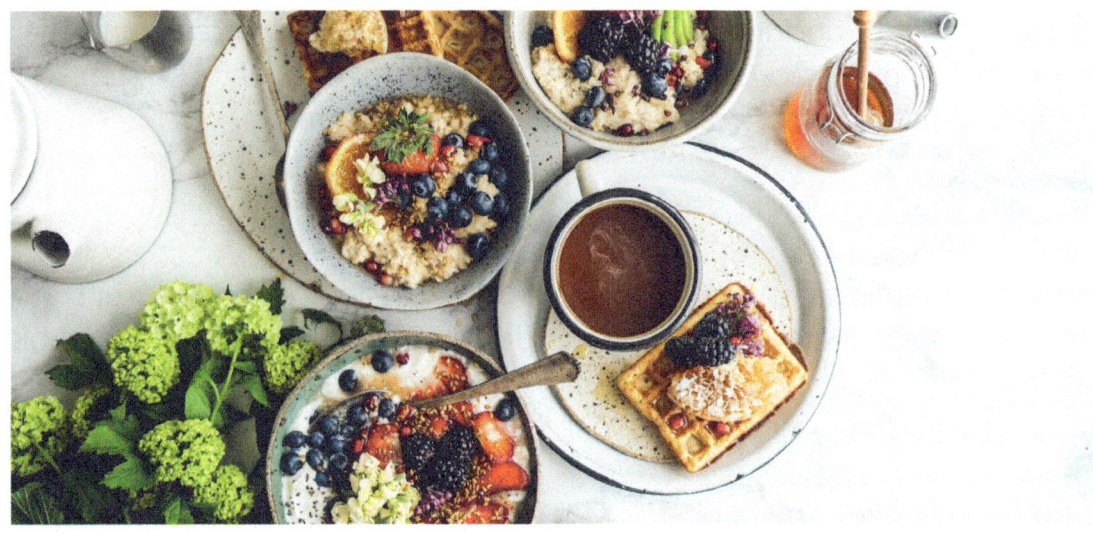

GIVE ME THE KEYS TO A TASTY NEW WAY OF LIFE

This cookbook isn't a treatment plan or a miracle cure. It's a collection of carefully crafted, tried and tested, nutritional and delicious recipes that will take the guesswork out of your new way of life. Because let's face it, Crohn's is here to stay.

So, you might as well use your chronic condition to create a new and beautiful lifestyle that will nurture and heal your body from the inside out. So, say goodbye to the things that weren't making you feel good anyway—the unhealthy, not particularly tasty meals accompanied by maybe a little too much alcohol or sugar or overly rich ingredients that your body struggled to process.

The goal has shifted, and now we're focused on eating to feel good with nutrient-rich, savory foods that your body can easily digest. Foods that will promote healing and soothing, and will deliver what your body needs to not only function properly but also feel great.

The recipes in this cookbook are affordable, simple, and easily modifiable. The dishes are both interesting and well-balanced. We can't have your tastebuds getting bored, after all! Living with Crohn's disease isn't a life sentence restricting you to bland food.

On the contrary, it's a reason to look within these pages and find all the foods you need to start eating as a gateway to a better way of living. With this book, you have everything you need to make a positive change in how you nourish your body and mind.

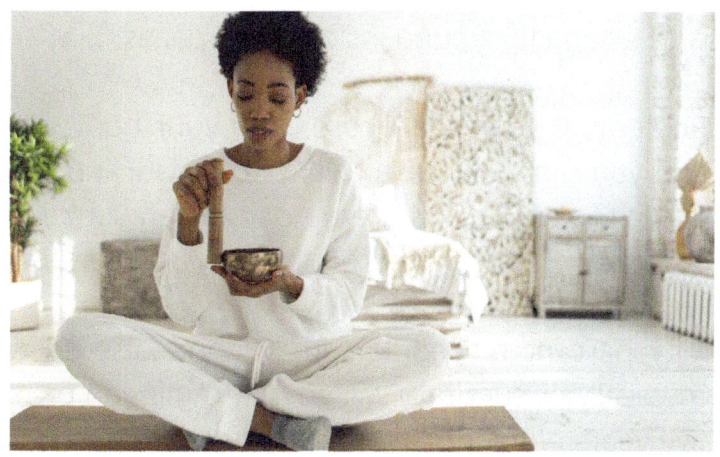

Look at it this way—Crohn's disease is something that you will have for the rest of your life, so why not get comfortable with the idea of healing yourself to a place of remission, and staying there for as long as possible?

Use this book as a tool to help you figure out what your body can and can't tolerate when you're in remission. Then, when you have a flare-up, you'll know just how to handle it.

Find the recipes that you absolutely adore and tweak the ones that aren't totally you by using alternatives to change things up a bit. You can always find delicious alternatives!

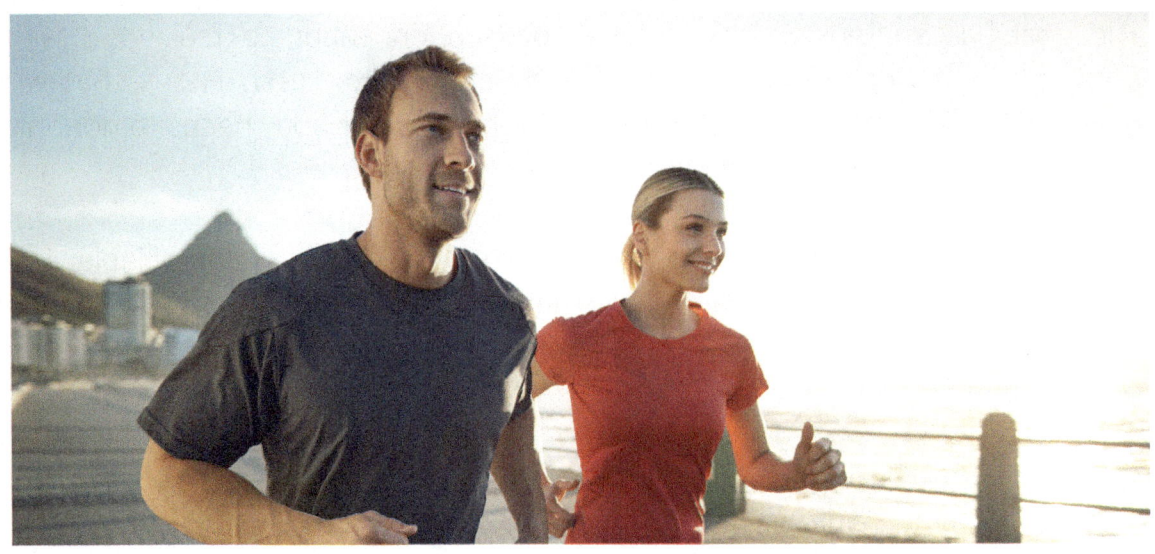

The recipes and menu plans in this book will make your flare-ups fewer and less severe. In no time at all, you'll know how to meet all your needs by using the recipes and tips found inside these pages.

Remember your goals here: heal your body, reduce your flare-ups, and know that you can continue to live a wonderful and healthy life without letting Crohn's get in the way. Will there be days when you're not feeling up to par? Sure. But you can do a lot to ensure those days are fewer and farther between.

Fifty percent of people with Crohn's disease who treat the condition either medically or surgically will go into remission or have only mild symptoms within five years of their diagnosis. Just think of how much higher you can boost those odds when you decide to give your body all the right nutrients, along with a little extra love in avoiding triggers that inflame it.

Follow the suggestions and recipes in this book, and see how much your body will benefit from the tasty fuel you feed it to start healing and maintaining itself.

Time to get started—you've got a delicious new life ahead!

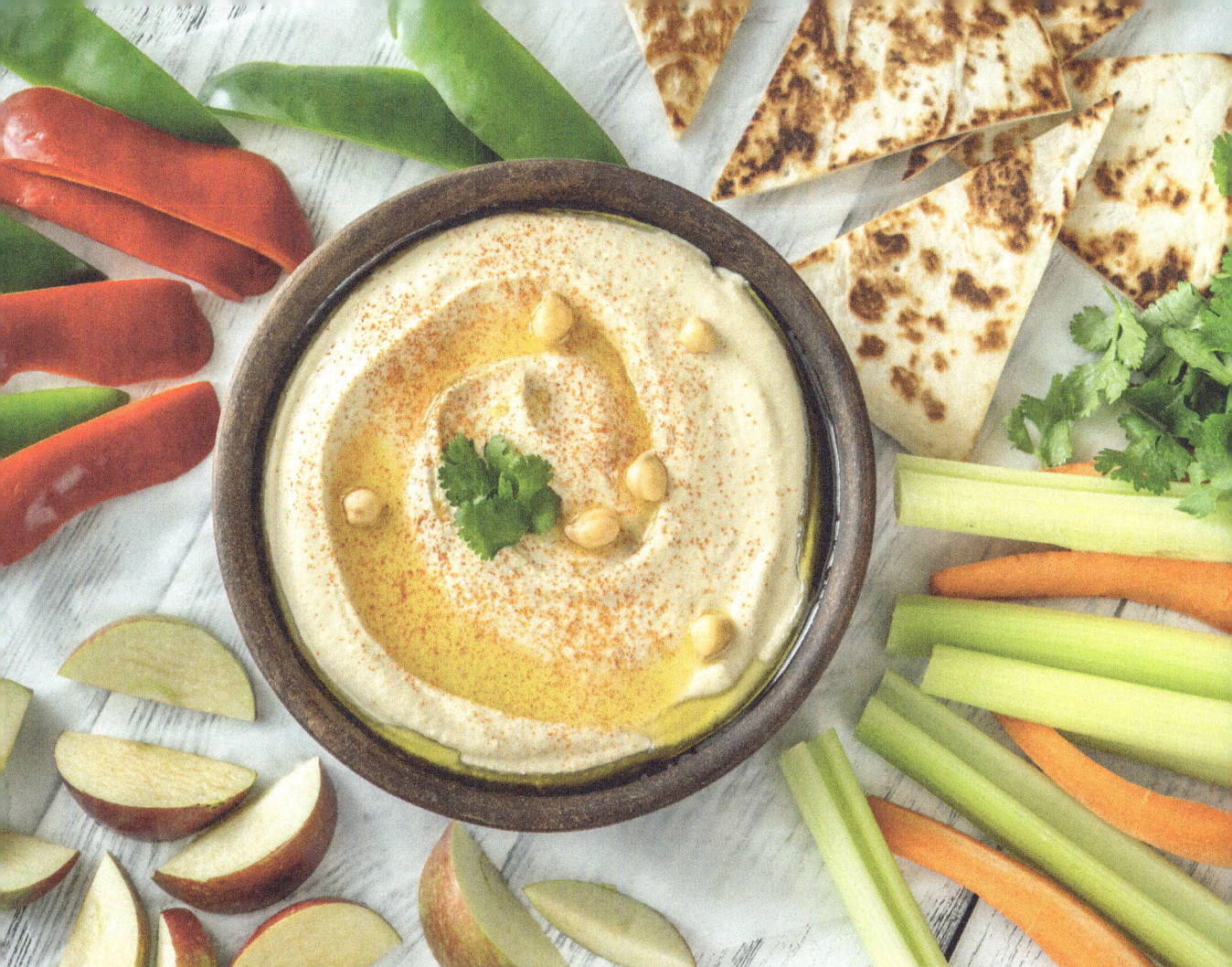

CHAPTER TWO: SNACKS

ROASTED CHICKPEAS

Ingredients:
- 1 can chickpeas
- 1 tbsp. olive oil
- 1 tsp. garlic powder
- 1/2 tsp. cumin
- 1/4 tsp. salt

Instructions:
1. Preheat oven to 400 degrees Fahrenheit.
2. Drain and rinse chickpeas.
3. Pat dry with a paper towel.
4. In a bowl, mix together olive oil, garlic powder, cumin, and salt.
5. Add chickpeas and toss to coat evenly.
6. Spread on a baking sheet and roast for 20-25 minutes until crispy.

Serving size: 1/2 cup
Calories: 100

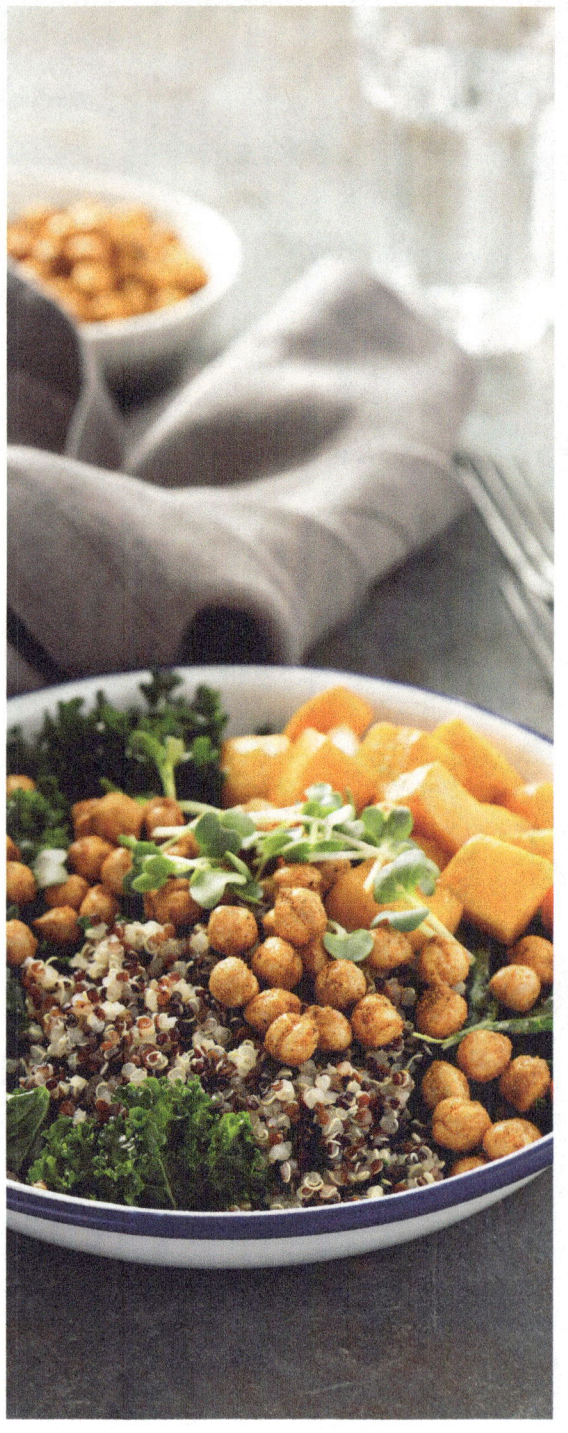

FRUIT AND NUT BARS

Ingredients:
- 1 cup dates
- 1/2 cup almonds
- 1/2 cup cashews
- 1/4 cup dried cranberries
- 1/4 cup desiccated coconut flakes

Instructions:
1. Place dates in a food processor and pulse until broken down.
2. Add almonds, cashews, cranberries, and coconut flakes.
3. Pulse until everything is finely chopped and well combined.
4. Line an 8x8 inch baking dish with parchment paper.
5. Transfer the mixture to the dish and press down firmly.
6. Place in the fridge for 30 minutes to set.
7. Cut into bars and enjoy!

Serving size: 1 bar
Calories: 180

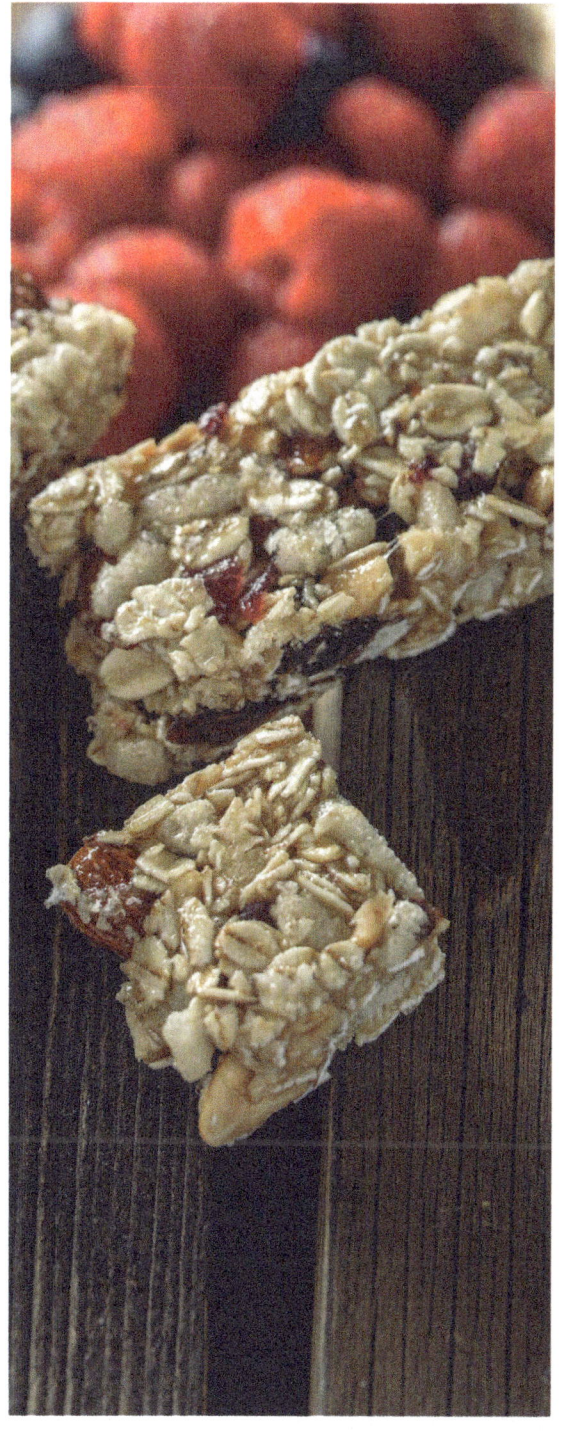

CUCUMBER AVOCADO TEA SANDWICHES

Ingredients:
- 4 slices gluten-free bread
- 1/2 cucumber
- 1/2 avocado
- 1 tbsp. lemon juice
- Salt and pepper to taste

Instructions:
1. Slice cucumber and avocado into thin pieces.
2. In a bowl, mix together lemon juice, salt, and pepper.
3. Toast bread slices.
4. Spread avocado on one slice and top with cucumber slices.
5. Drizzle with the lemon juice mixture.
6. Top with another slice of toast.
7. Cut into four pieces and serve immediately.

Serving size: 1 sandwich
Calories: 220

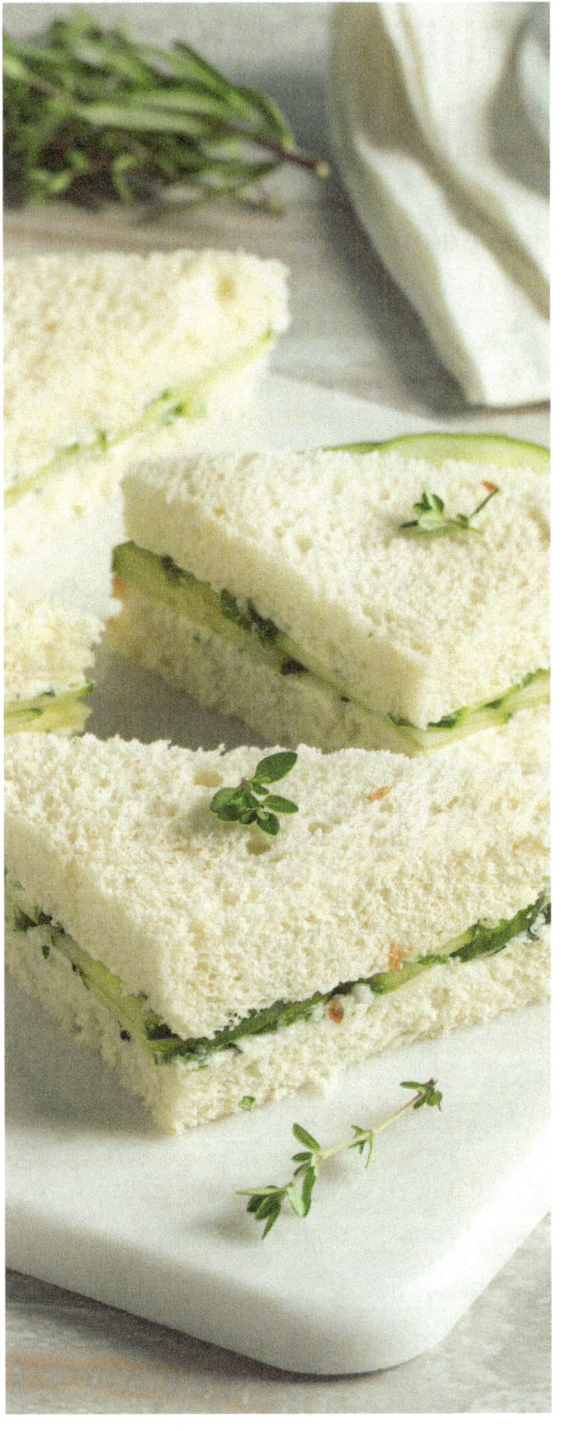

CHOCOLATE HUMMUS

Ingredients:
- 1 can chickpeas
- 1/4 cup cocoa powder
- 1/4 cup agave nectar
- 1 tbsp. olive oil
- 2 tsp. vanilla extract
- 1/4 tsp. salt

Instructions:
1. Drain and rinse chickpeas.
2. Pat dry with a paper towel.
3. In a food processor, combine chickpeas, cocoa powder, agave nectar, olive oil, vanilla extract, and salt.
4. Blend until smooth.
5. Serve with fruit, pretzels, or graham crackers for dipping.

Serving size: 2 tbsp.
Calories: 80

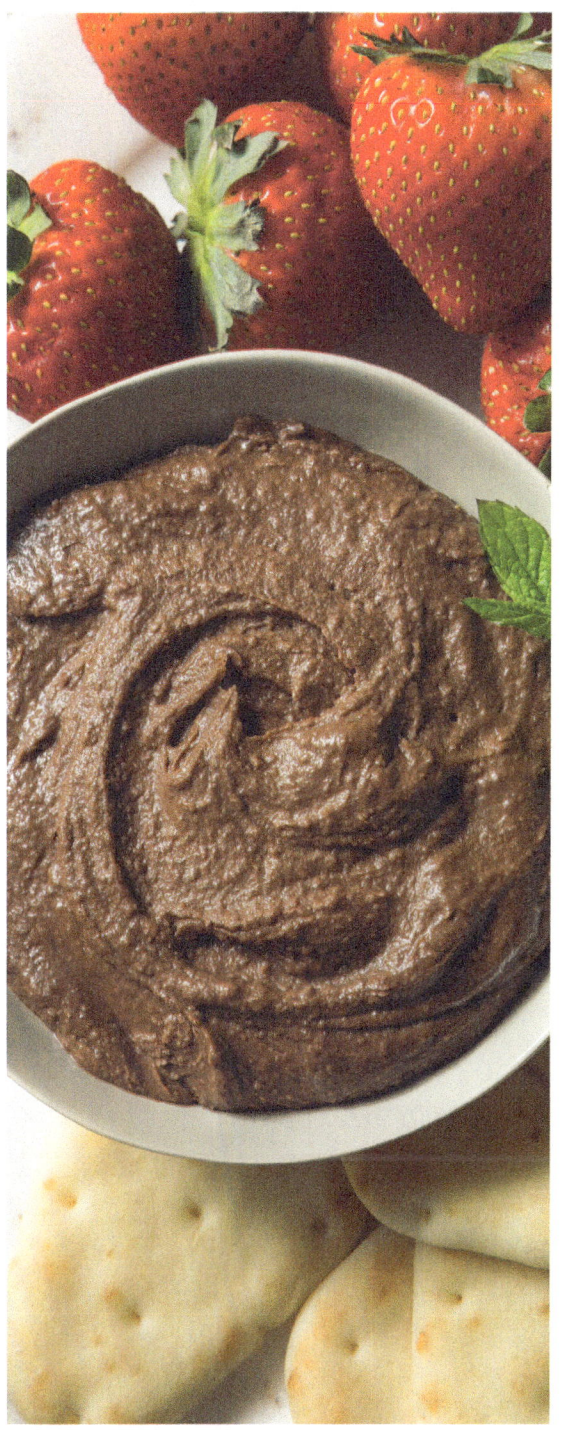

SWEET POTATO CHIPS

Ingredients:
- 1 large sweet potato
- 1 tbsp. olive oil
- salt and pepper to taste

Instructions:
1. Preheat oven to 400 degrees Fahrenheit.
2. Line a baking sheet with parchment paper.
3. Slice sweet potato into thin rounds.
4. In a bowl, toss sweet potato slices with olive oil and salt and pepper.
5. Spread on the prepared baking sheet and bake for 20-25 minutes until crispy.
6. Let cool before serving.

Serving size: 1/2 cup
Calories: 100

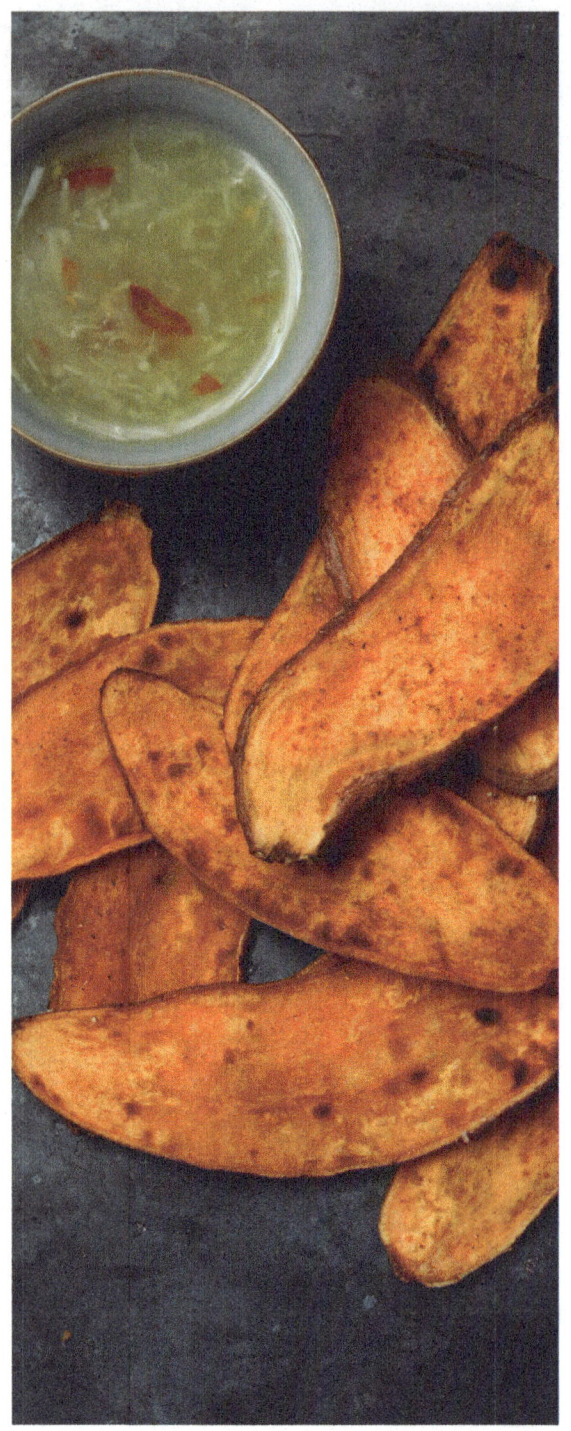

PARMESAN GARLIC KALE CHIPS

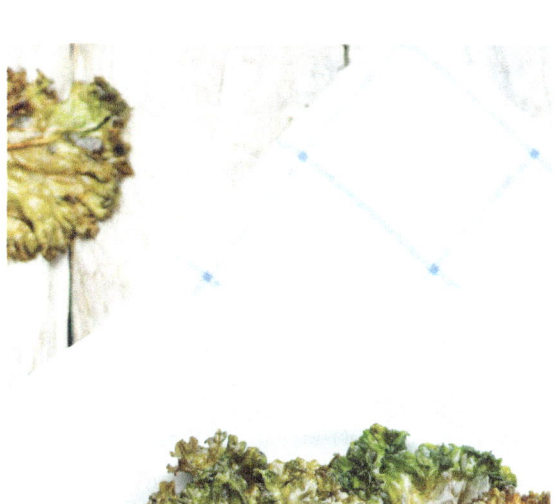

Ingredients:
- 1 bunch kale
- 1/4 cup grated Parmesan cheese
- 1 tbsp. olive oil
- 1 tsp. garlic powder
- 1/4 tsp. salt

Instructions:
1. Preheat oven to 375 degrees Fahrenheit.
2. Line a baking sheet with parchment paper.
3. Remove the kale from the stem and tear into bite-sized pieces.
4. In a bowl, mix together Parmesan cheese, olive oil, garlic powder, and salt.
5. Add the kale and toss to coat evenly.
6. Spread on the prepared baking sheet and bake for 10-15 minutes until crispy.

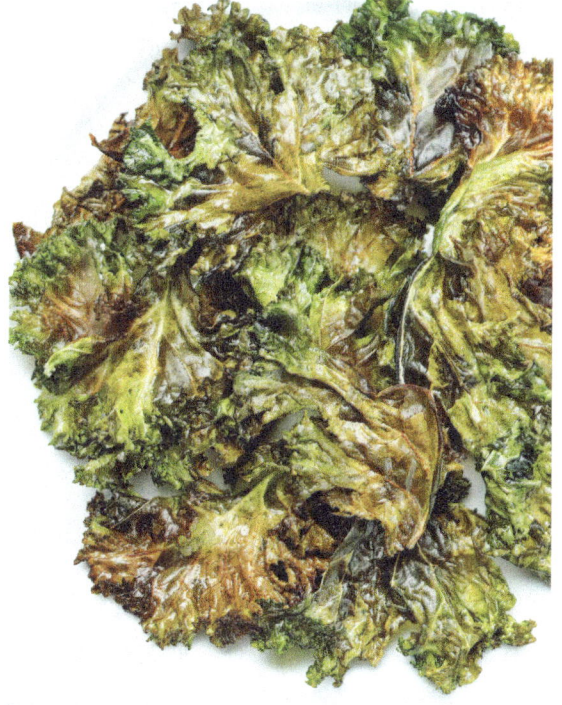

Serving size: 1/2 cup
Calories: 80

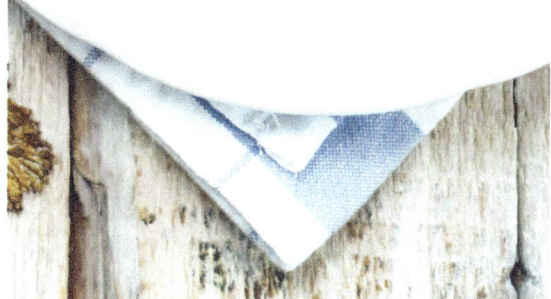

SPICY ROASTED EDAMAME

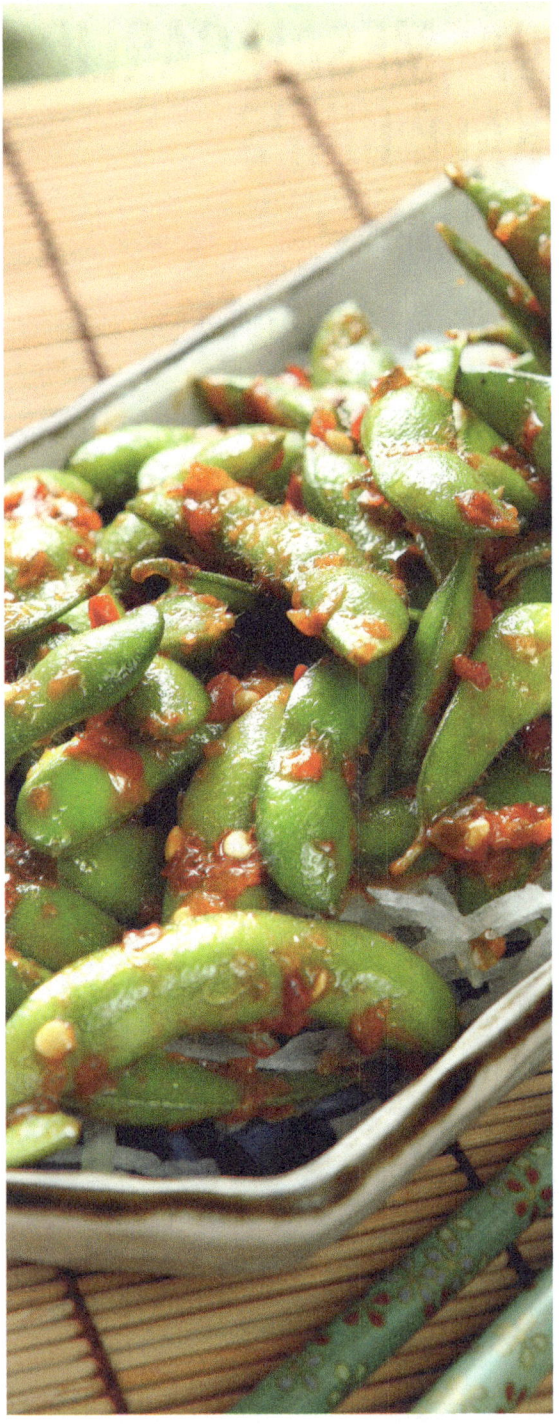

Ingredients:
- 1 lb. edamame in the shell
- 1 tablespoon olive oil
- 1 teaspoon chili powder
- 1 teaspoon smoked paprika
- 1/2 teaspoon garlic powder
- 1/4 teaspoon salt

Instructions:
1. Preheat oven to 375 degrees F.
2. In a large bowl, combine edamame, olive oil, chili powder, smoked paprika, garlic powder, and salt.
3. Toss to coat evenly.
4. Spread edamame in a single layer on a baking sheet.
5. Roast for about 15-20 minutes, or until slightly browned and crisp.
6. Remove from oven and let cool slightly.
7. Serve warm and enjoy!

Serving size: 4 people
Calories: 100 calories

TRAIL MIX

Ingredients:
- 1/2 cup almonds
- 1/2 cup cashews
- 1/2 cup dried cranberries
- 1/4 cup chocolate chips.

Instructions:
1. Place all ingredients in a bowl and mix together.
2. Enjoy as is or pack into individual bags for on-the-go snacking.

Serving size: 1/4 cup
Calories: 160

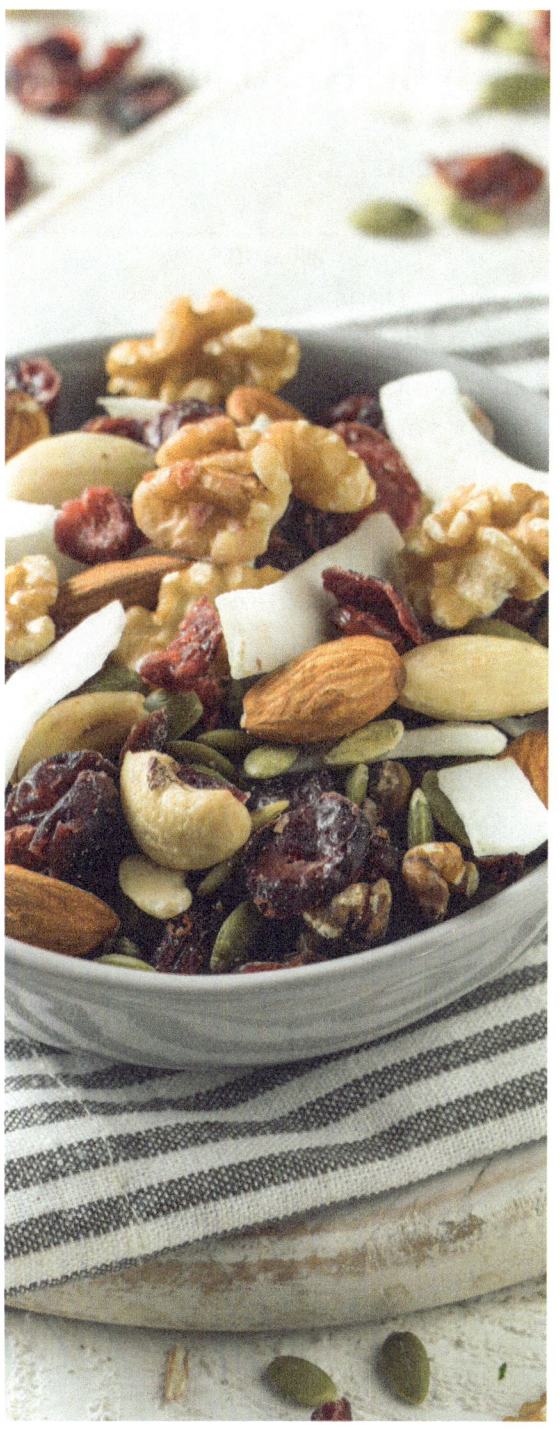

BANANA SUSHI

Ingredients:
- 2 bananas
- 1 tbsp. peanut butter
- 2 tsp. Honey
- 4 dates
- 1/4 cup unsweetened shredded coconut

Instructions:
1. Peel bananas and cut into thirds.
2. Spread peanut butter on top of each banana slice.
3. Place dates on a cutting board and chop into small pieces.
4. Sprinkle over the peanut butter.
5. Roll up each banana slice and then coat in shredded coconut.
6. Serve immediately.

Serving size: 1 roll
Calories: 150

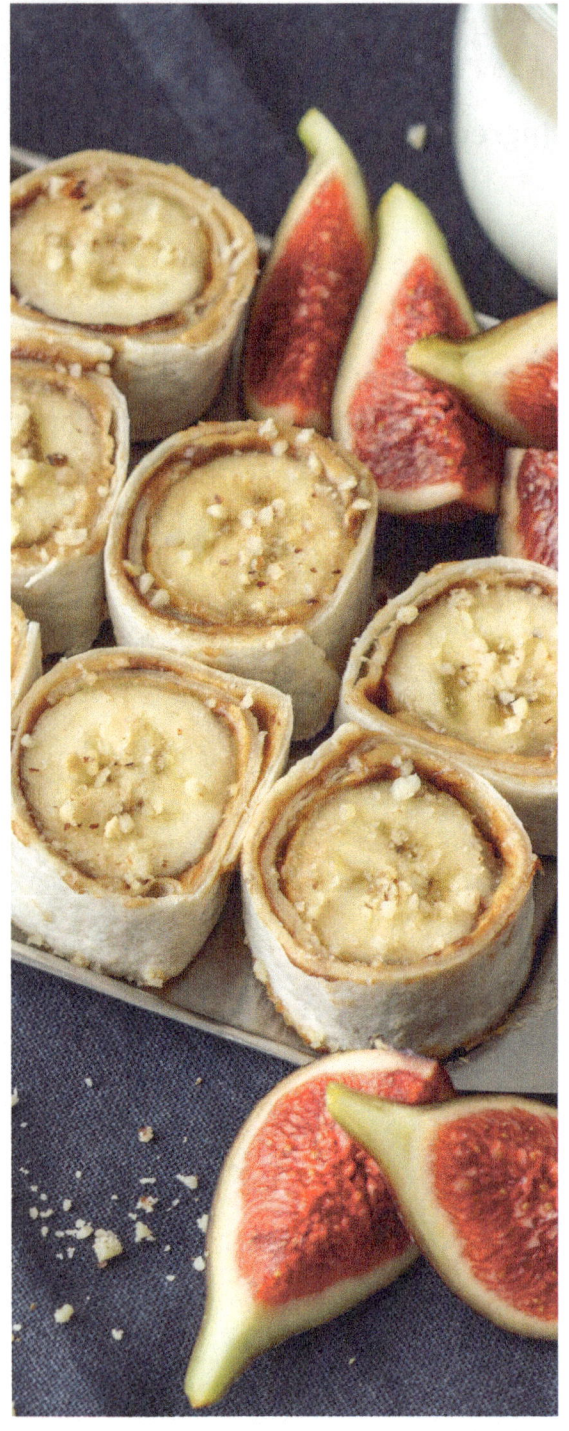

APPLE NACHOS

Ingredients:
- 1 apple
- 1 tbsp. peanut butter
- 2 tsp. honey, 4 dates
- 1/4 cup unsweetened shredded coconut flakes

Instructions:
1. Cut apple into thin slices.
2. Spread peanut butter on top of each slice.
3. Place dates on a cutting board and chop into small pieces.
4. Sprinkle over the peanut butter.
5. Top with shredded coconut flakes.
6. Serve immediately.

Serving size: 1 apple slice
Calories: 80

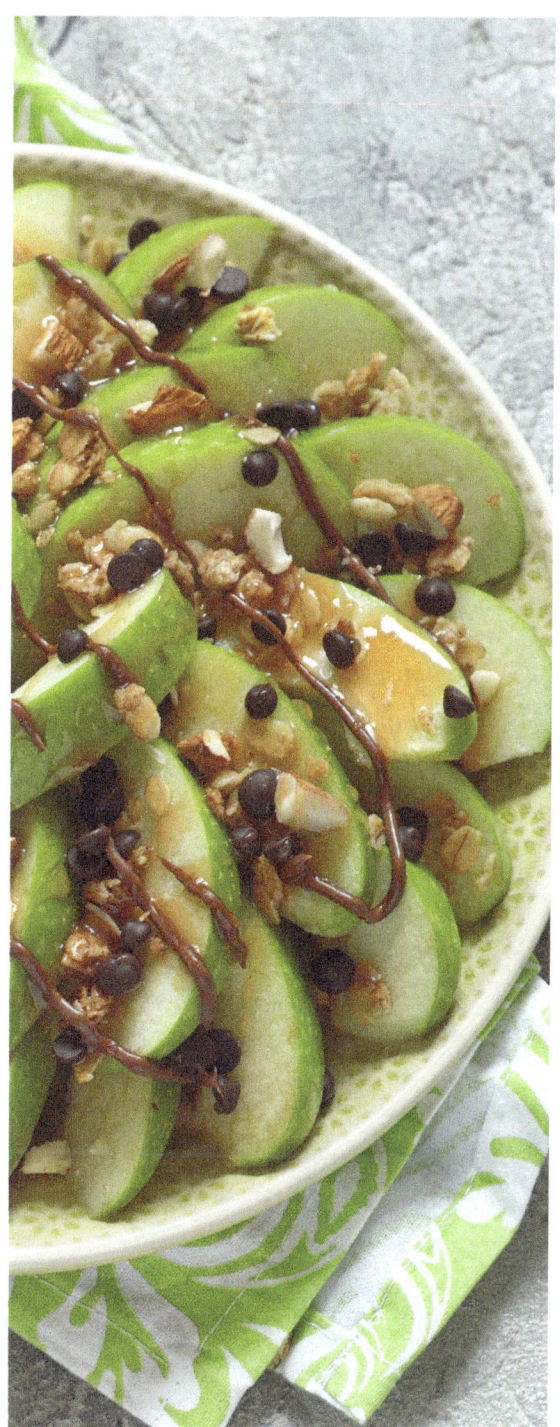

CUCUMBER BITES

Ingredients:
- 1 English cucumber
- 1/4 cup plain Greek yogurt
- 2 tbsp. sriracha sauce
- 1 tsp. Honey
- 1/4 tsp. salt
- 1/4 tsp. pepper
- 1/4 cup chopped fresh cilantro

Instructions:
1. Slice cucumber into bite-sized pieces.
2. In a small bowl, mix together Greek yogurt, sriracha sauce, honey, salt and pepper.
3. Spoon the mixture onto the cucumber slices and top with fresh cilantro.
4. Serve immediately.

Serving size: 2 cucumber bites
Calories: 50

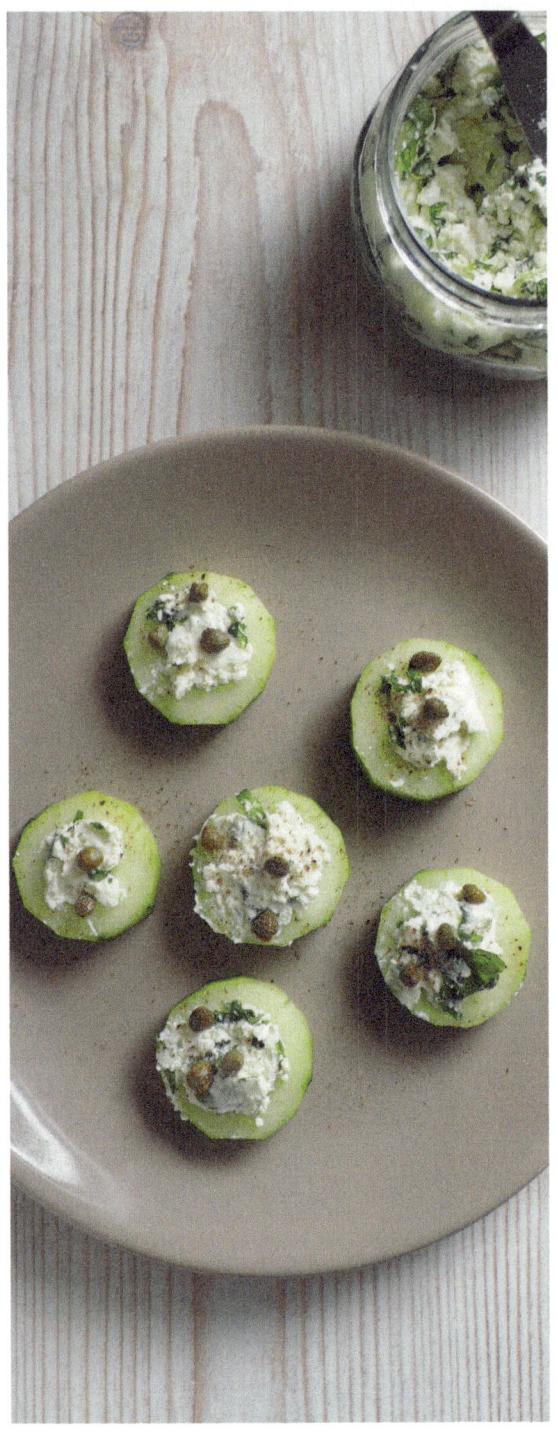

CHERRY TOMATOES WITH BASIL

Ingredients:
- 1 pint cherry tomatoes
- 2 tbsp. chopped fresh basil
- 1 tsp. balsamic vinegar
- 1/4 tsp. Salt
- 1/4 tsp. Pepper

Instructions:
1. Place cherry tomatoes in a bowl.
2. Add chopped basil, balsamic vinegar, salt and pepper.
3. Toss to coat evenly. Serve immediately or store in the fridge for later.
4. Enjoy!

Serving size: 1/2 cup
Calories: 50

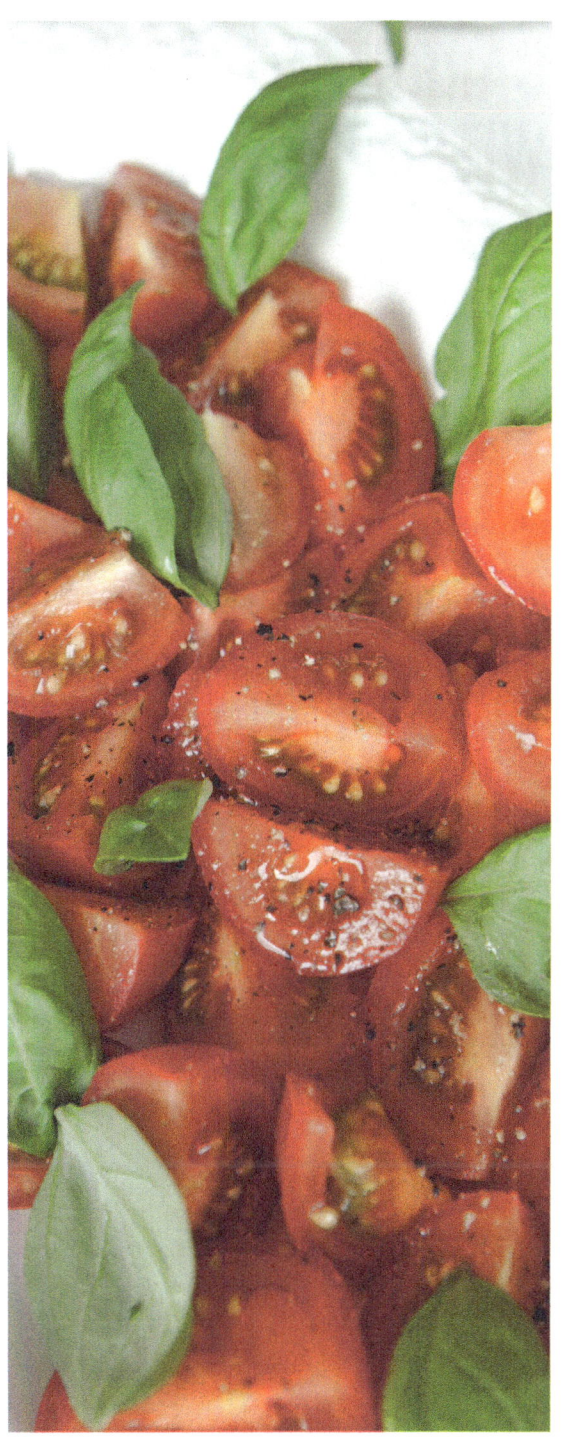

CARROT STICKS WITH HUMMUS

Ingredients:
- 1 lb. carrots
- 1 cup prepared hummus
- 2 tbsp. freshly squeezed lemon juice
- 1/4 tsp. Cumin
- salt and pepper to taste

Instructions:
1. Cut carrots into sticks.
2. In a small bowl, mix together hummus, lemon juice, cumin, salt and pepper.
3. Serve the carrot sticks with the hummus dip.

Serving size: 1/2 cup
Calories: 100

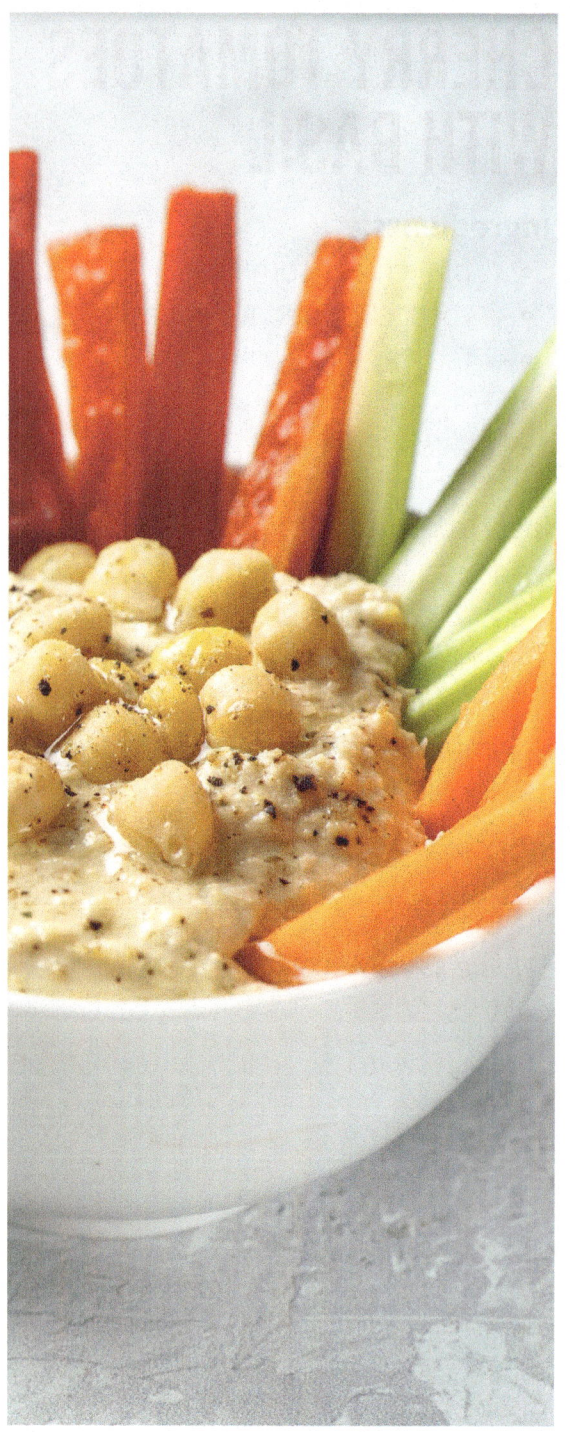

CELERY STICKS WITH PEANUT BUTTER

Ingredients:
- 1 lb. celery
- 1/2 cup natural peanut butter
- 2 tbsp. Honey
- 1/4 tsp. Salt

Instructions:
1. Cut celery into sticks.
2. In a small bowl, mix together peanut butter, honey and salt.
3. Serve the celery sticks with the peanut butter dip.

Serving size: 1/2 cup
Calories: 150

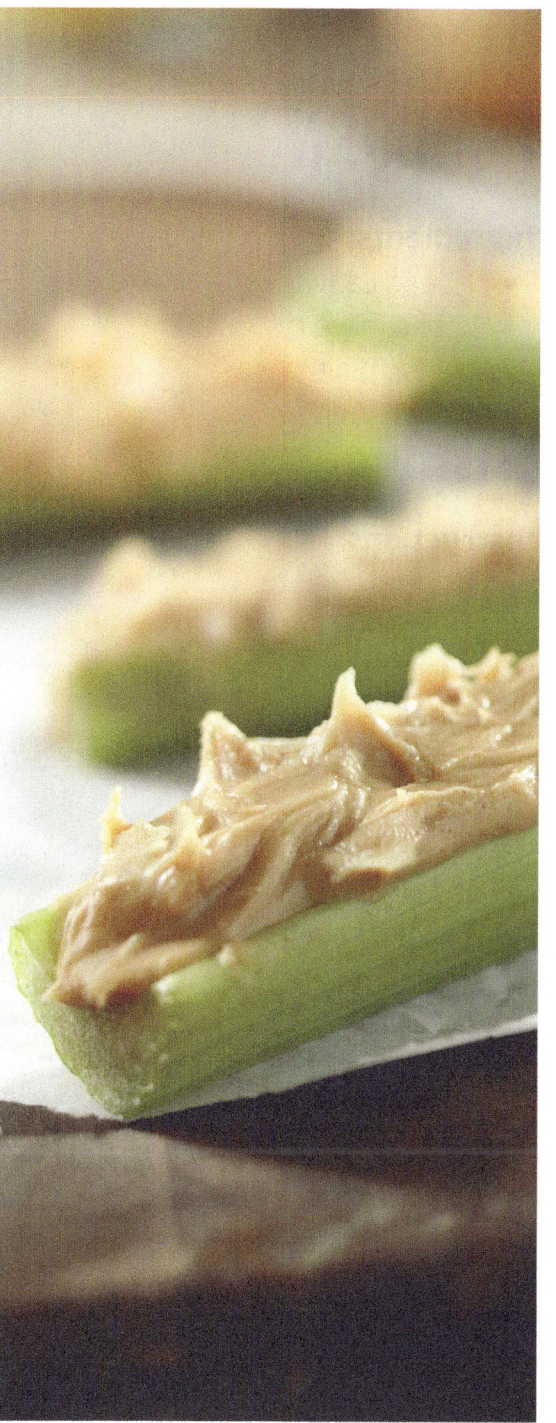

CAULIFLOWER POPCORN

Ingredients:
- 1 head cauliflower
- 2 tbsp. olive oil
- 1/4 tsp. Salt
- 1/4 tsp. pepper
- 1/4 cup grated Parmesan cheese

Instructions:
1. Preheat oven to 375 degrees Fahrenheit.
2. Line a baking sheet with parchment paper.
3. Cut cauliflower into small popcorn-sized pieces.
4. In a bowl, mix together olive oil, salt and pepper.
5. Add the cauliflower and toss to coat evenly.
6. Spread on the prepared baking sheet and bake for 25-30 minutes until golden brown and crispy.
7. Remove from the oven and sprinkle with Parmesan cheese.
8. Serve immediately.

Serving size: 1/2 cup
Calories: 100

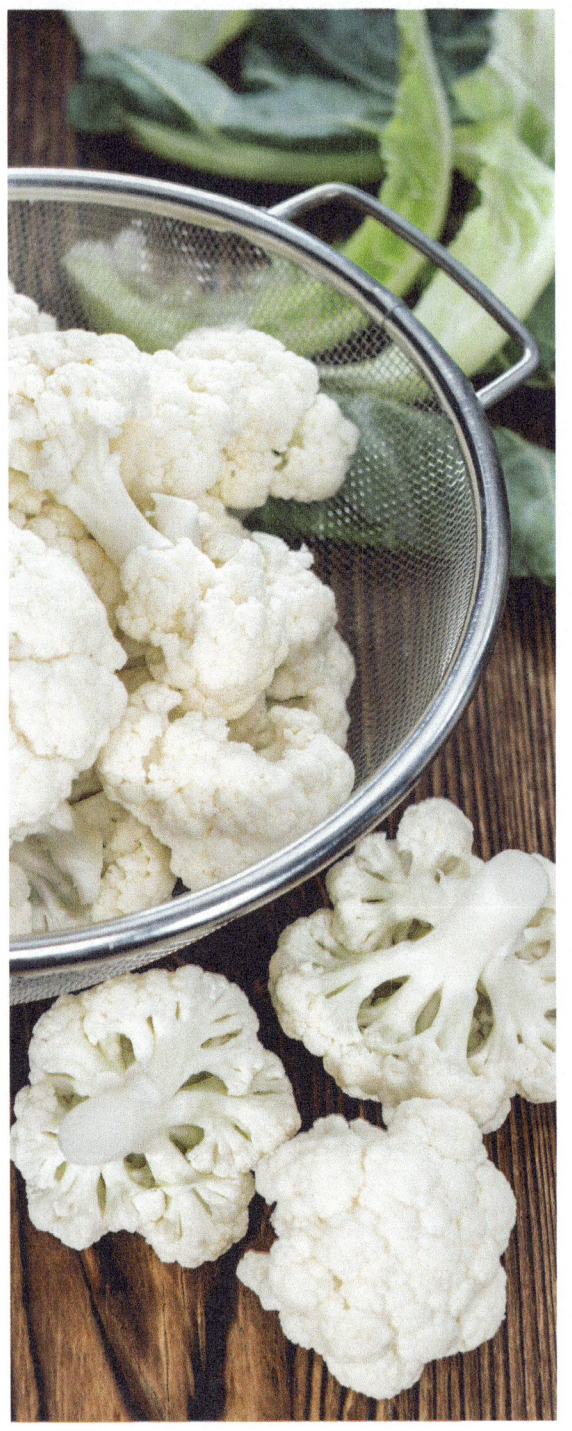

EDAMAME

Ingredients:
- 1 package frozen edamame
- 2 tbsp. soy sauce
- 1 tbsp. Honey
- 1 clove garlic minced

Instructions:
1. Cook edamame according to package directions.
2. In a small bowl, mix together soy sauce, honey and garlic.
3. Drain the edamame and add it to the bowl with the sauce.
4. Toss to coat evenly.
5. Serve immediately.

Serving size: 1/2 cup
Calories: 100

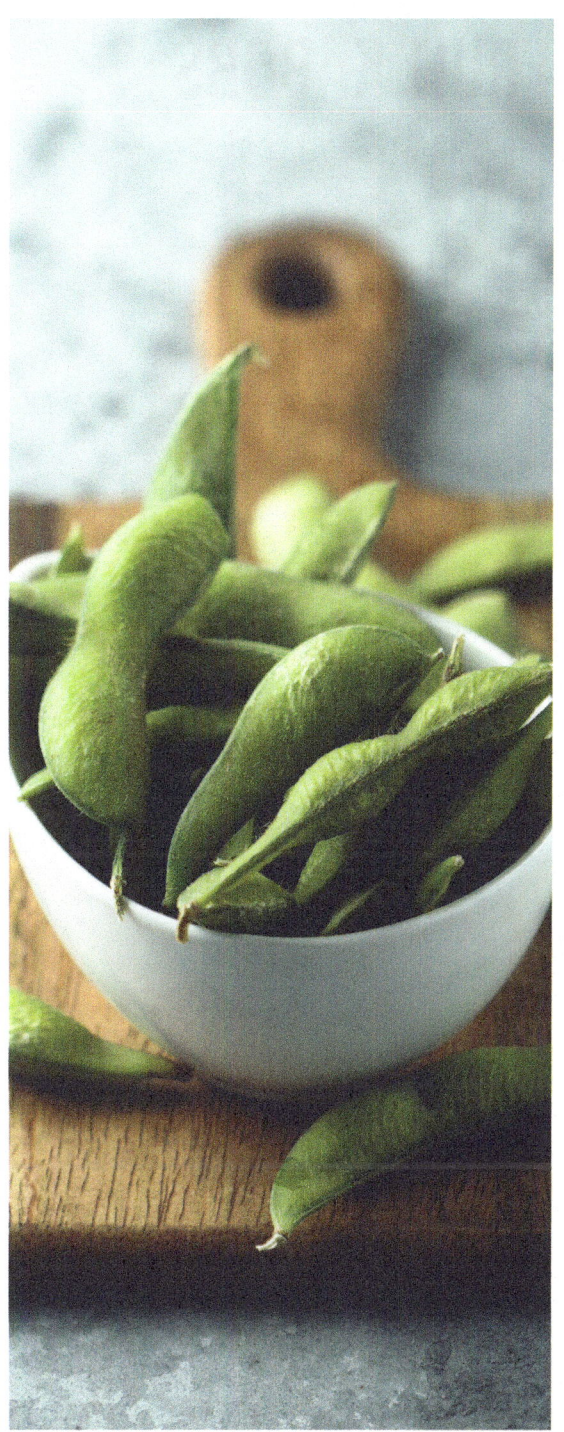

FRUIT KABOBS

Ingredients:
- 1 apple
- 1 pear
- 1 banana
- 1/4 cup raisins
- 2 tbsp. peanut butter
- 4 skewers

Instructions:
1. Cut fruit into bite-sized pieces.
2. Thread onto skewers alternating between fruit and raisins.
3. In a small bowl, mix together peanut butter and a few drops of water to thin.
4. Drizzle over the kabobs.
5. Enjoy!

Serving size: 1 kabob
Calories: 150

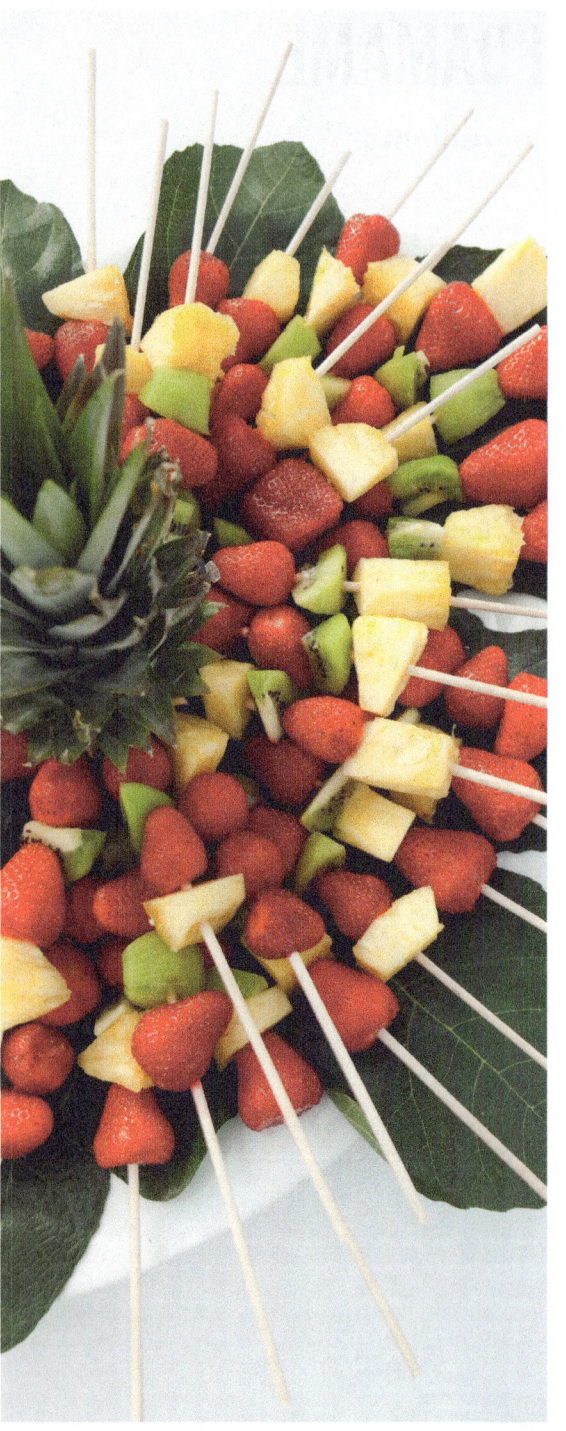

GRAPEFRUIT WITH HONEY

Ingredients:
- 1 grapefruit
- 2 tbsp. Honey
- 1/4 tsp. ground ginger

Instructions:
1. Cut grapefruit in half and spoon out the flesh into a bowl.
2. Add honey and ginger and mix together until well combined.
3. Enjoy!

Serving size: 1 grapefruit half
Calories: 100

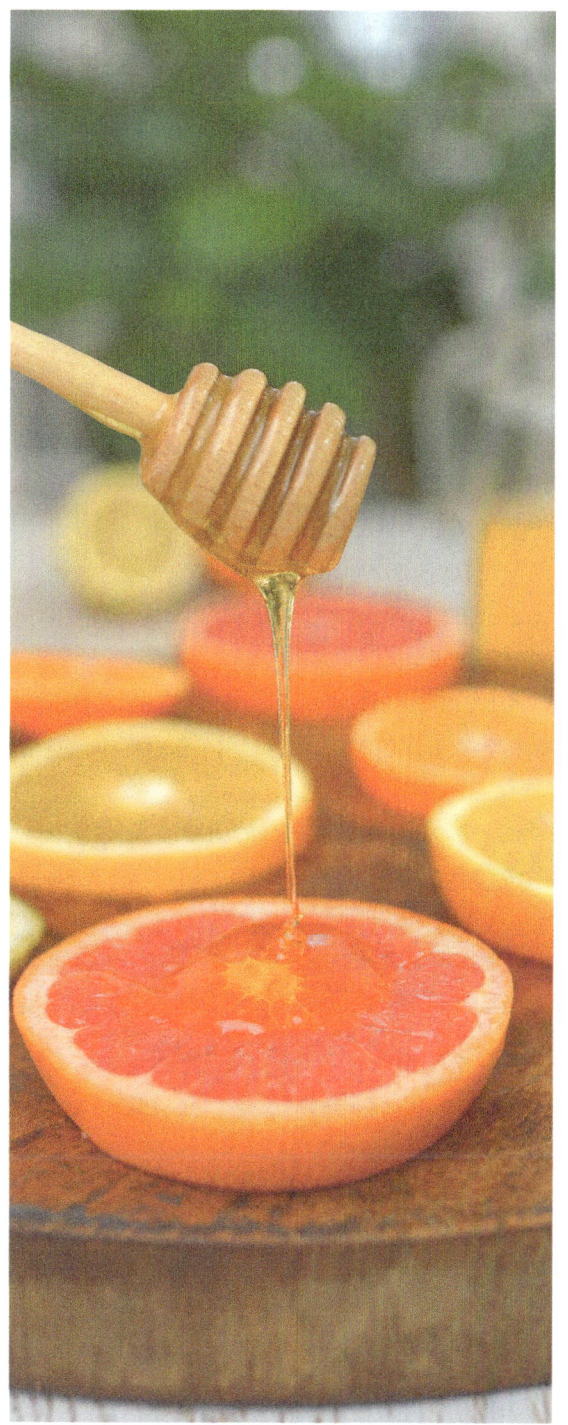

CANTALOUPE WITH COTTAGE CHEESE

Ingredients:
- 1/2 cantaloupe
- 1/2 cup cottage cheese
- 2 tbsp. Granola
- 1 tbsp. Honey

Instructions:
1. Scoop out the cantaloupe and add it to a bowl.
2. Add cottage cheese, granola and honey.
3. Mix together until well combined.

Serving size: 1/2 cantaloupe
Calories: 150

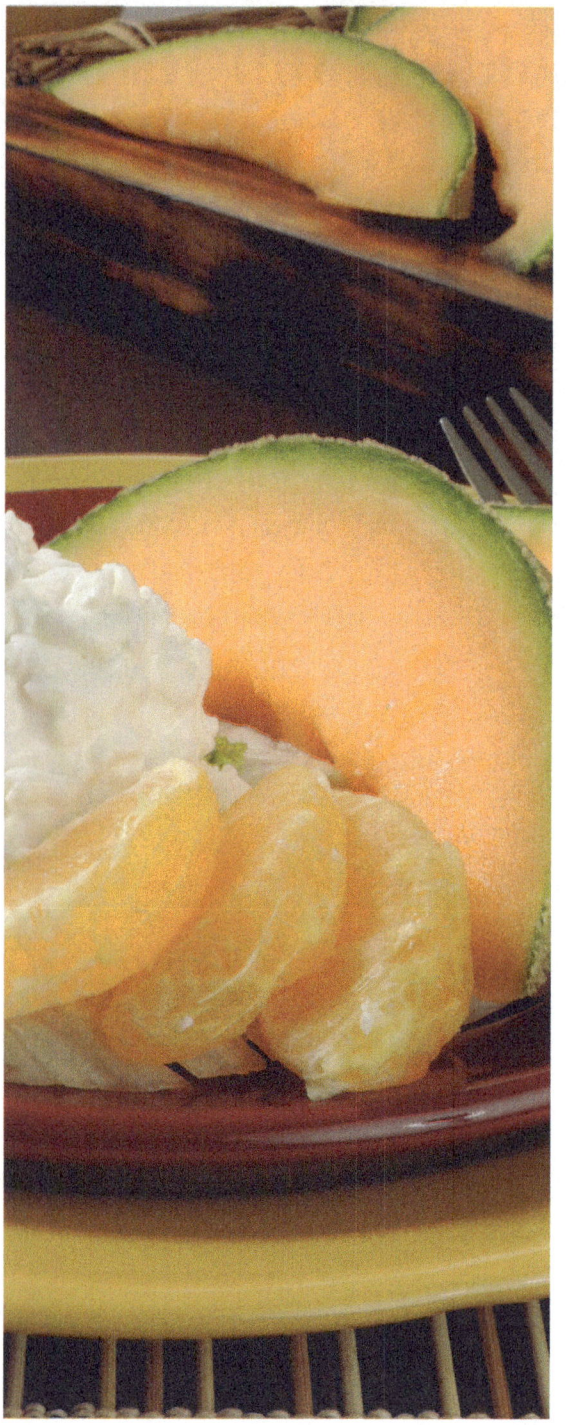

ORANGE WITH ALMOND BUTTER

Ingredients:
- 1 orange
- 2 tbsp. almond butter
- 1/4 tsp. ground cinnamon

Instructions:
1. Cut the top off of the orange and scoop out the flesh into a bowl.
2. Add almond butter and cinnamon and mix together until well combined.
3. Enjoy!

Serving size: 1 orange
Calories: 100

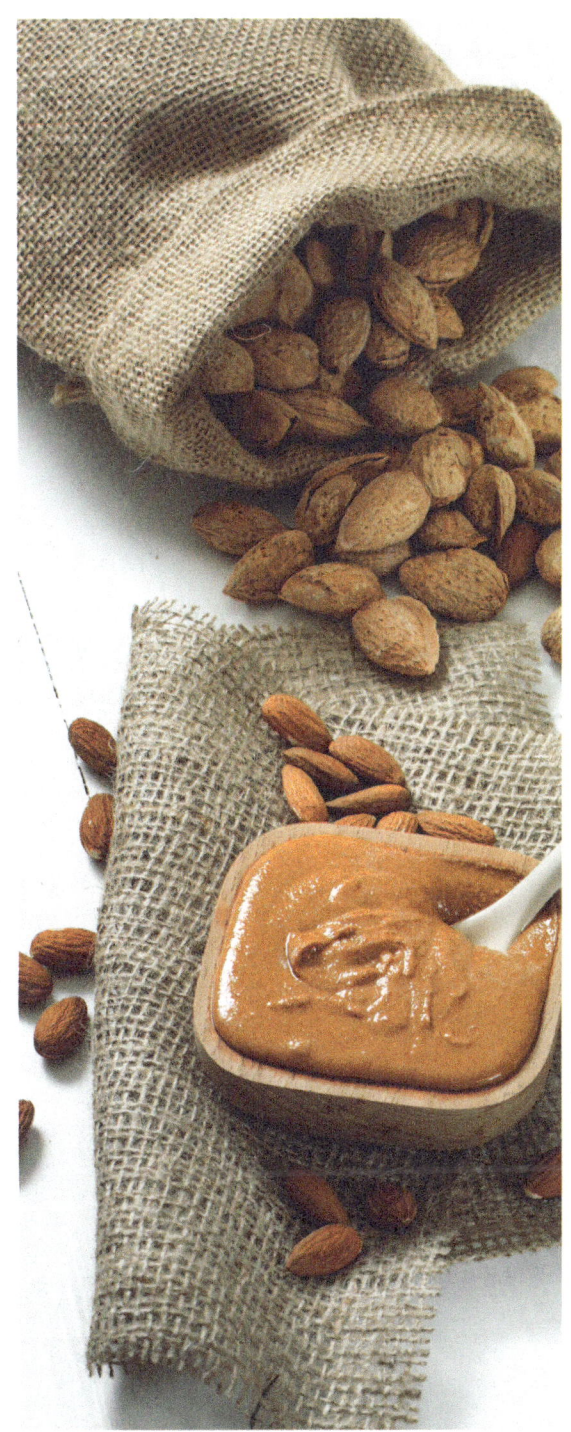

PEACH WITH YOGURT

Ingredients:
- 1 peach
- 1/2 cup yogurt
- 2 tbsp. Granola
- 1 tbsp. Honey

Instructions:
1. Cut the peach in half and remove the pit.
2. Add the peach halves to a bowl.
3. Add yogurt, granola and honey.
4. Mix together until well combined.

Serving size: 1 peach
Calories: 150

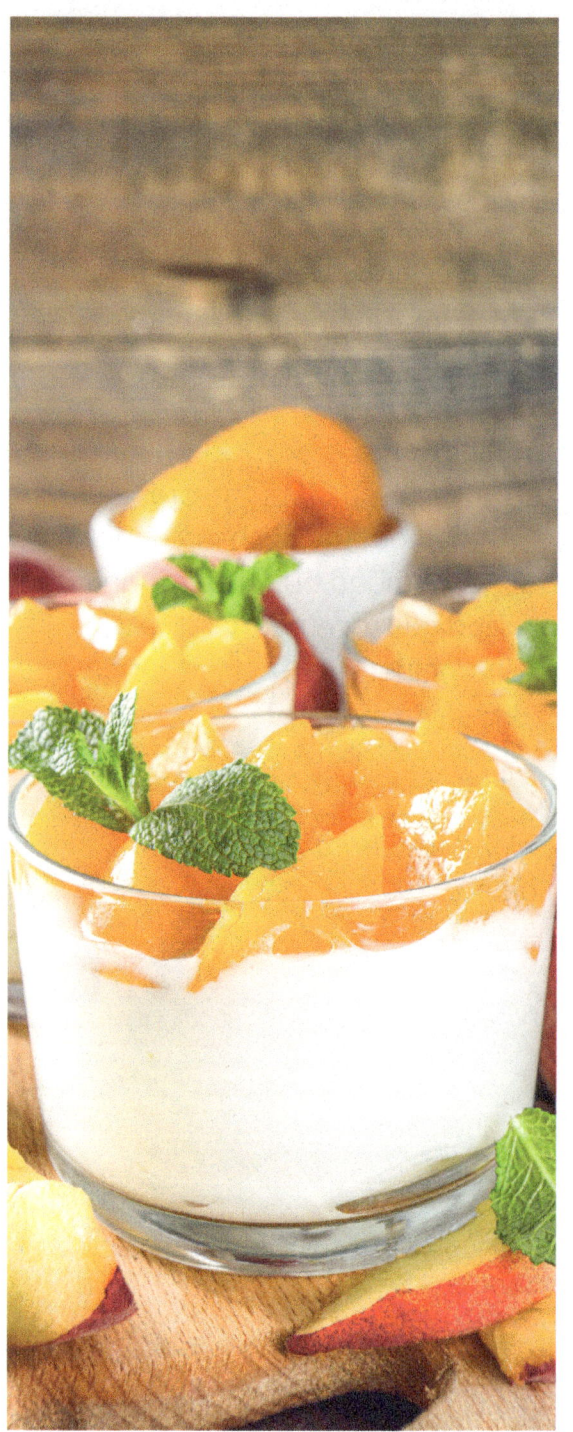

PINEAPPLE WITH COCONUT MILK

Ingredients:
- 1 cup pineapple
- 1/4 cup coconut milk
- 2 tbsp. Honey
- 1/4 tsp. ground ginger

Instructions:
1. 1. Add pineapple, coconut milk, honey and ginger to a blender and blend until smooth.
2. 2. Enjoy!

Serving size: 1 cup
Calories: 100

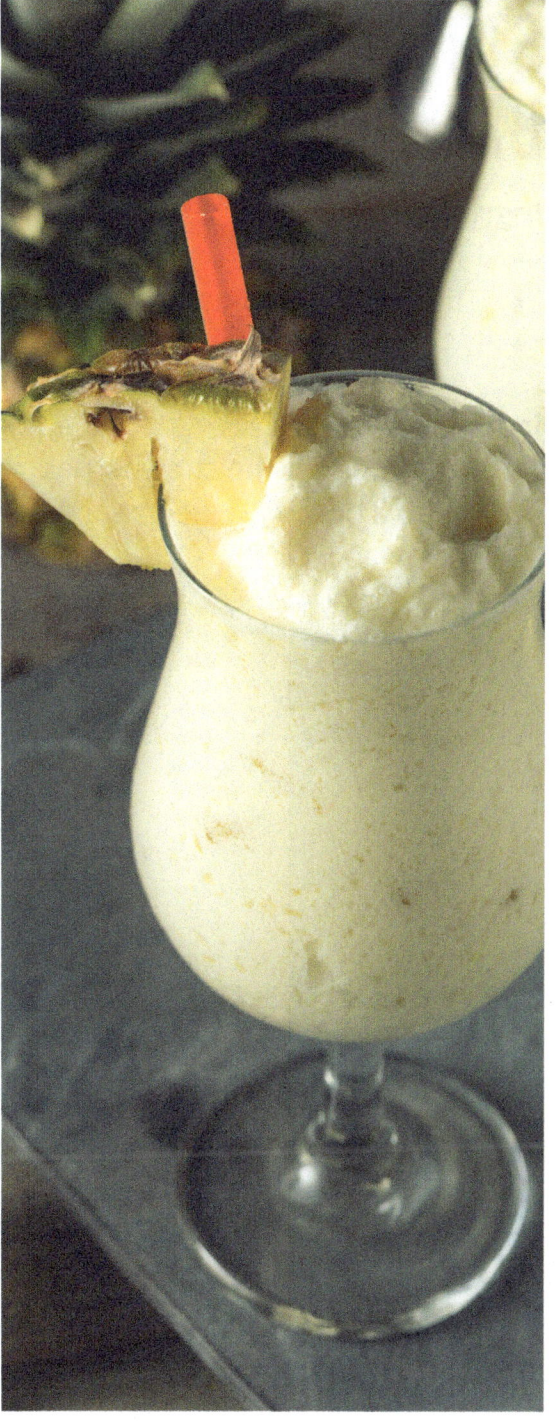

STRAWBERRY WITH BALSAMIC VINEGAR

Ingredients:
- 1 lb. strawberries
- 2 tbsp. balsamic vinegar
- 1/4 tsp. Salt

Instructions:
1. Wash and slice the strawberries.
2. Add to a bowl with the balsamic vinegar and salt.
3. Toss to coat evenly.

Serving size: 1 cup
Calories: 50

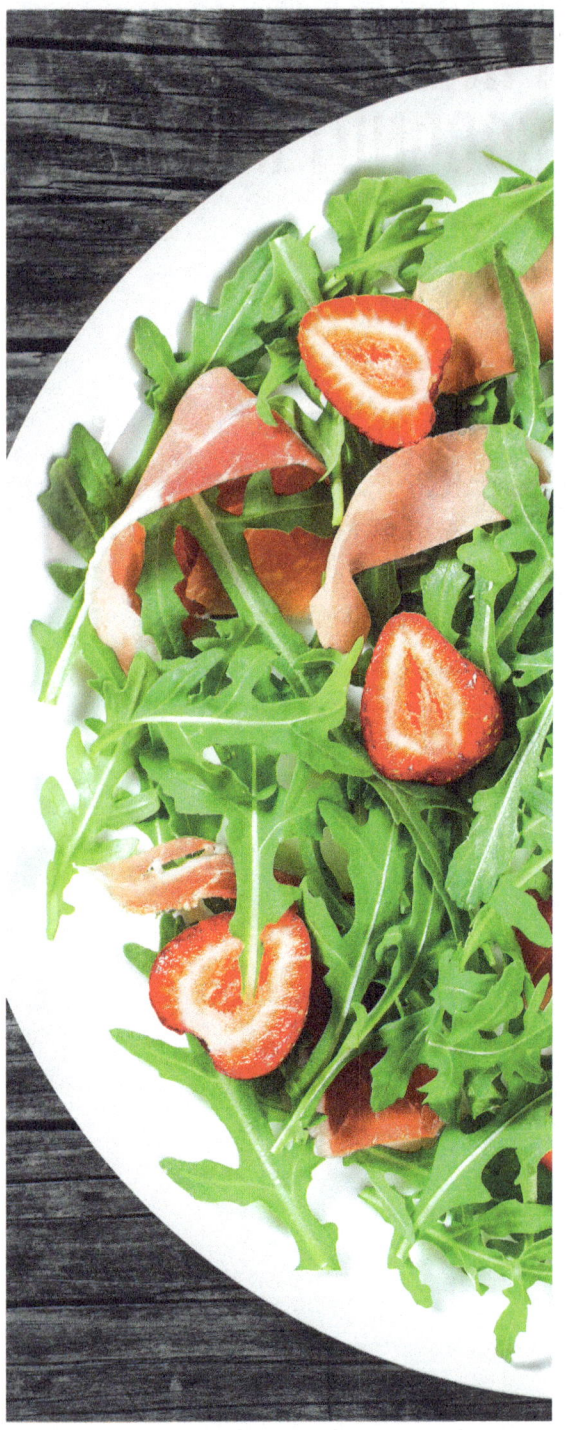

WATERMELON WITH MINT

Ingredients:
- 1 lb. watermelon
- 2 tbsp. Honey
- 1/4 tsp. ground ginger
- 1/4 cup chopped mint

Instructions:
1. Cut the watermelon into bite-sized pieces.
2. Add to a bowl with the honey, ginger and mint.
3. Mix together until well combined.
4. Enjoy!

Serving size: 1 cup
Calories: 50

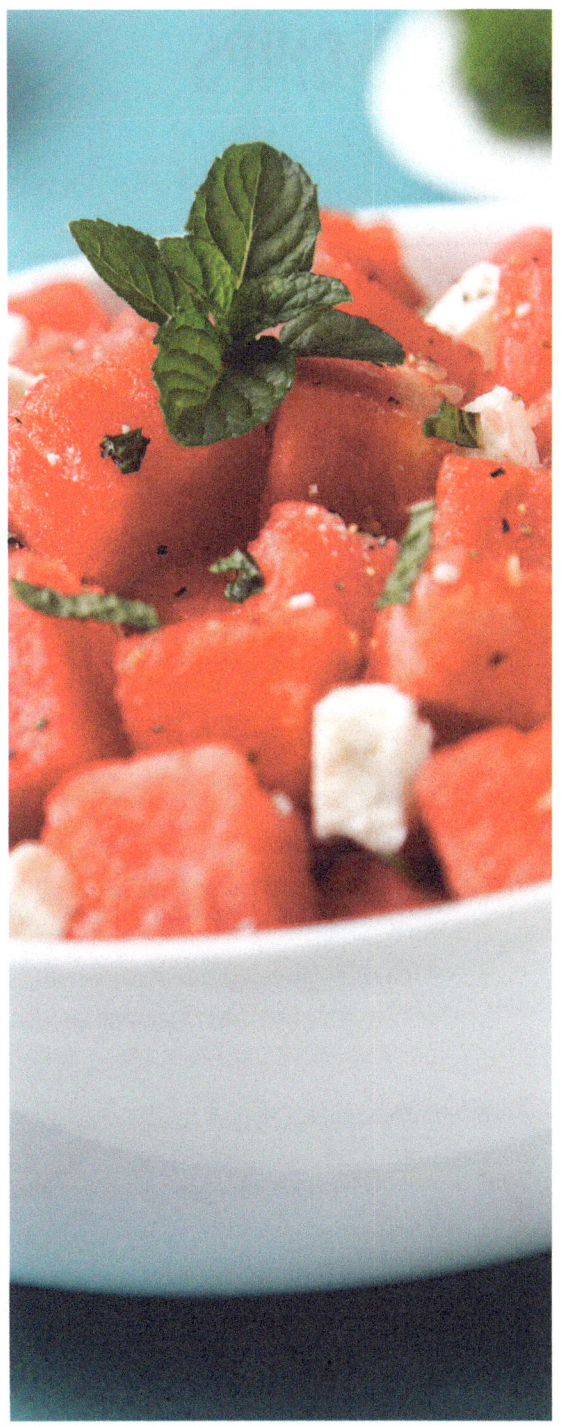

VEGGIE CHIPS

Ingredients:
- 1 large sweet potato, sliced into thin chips
- 1 small zucchini, sliced into thin chips
- 1 small yellow squash, sliced into thin chips
- 1 tablespoon olive oil
- 1/4 teaspoon salt

Instructions:
1. Preheat oven to 375 degrees F.
2. In a large bowl, combine sweet potato slices, zucchini slices, and yellow squash slices.
3. Drizzle with olive oil and season with salt. Toss to coat evenly.
4. Spread veggies in a single layer on a baking sheet.
5. Bake for about 20-25 minutes, or until chips are golden brown and crisp.
6. Remove from oven and let cool slightly.
7. Serve warm and enjoy!

Serving size: 4 people
Calories: 100 calories

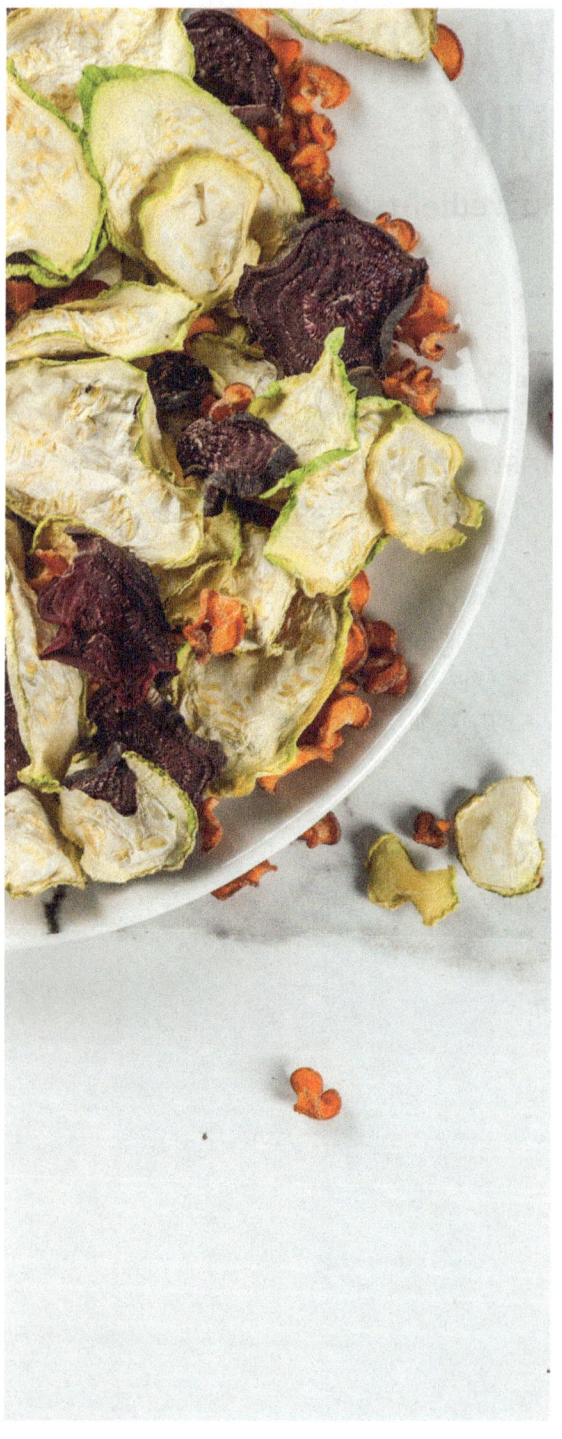

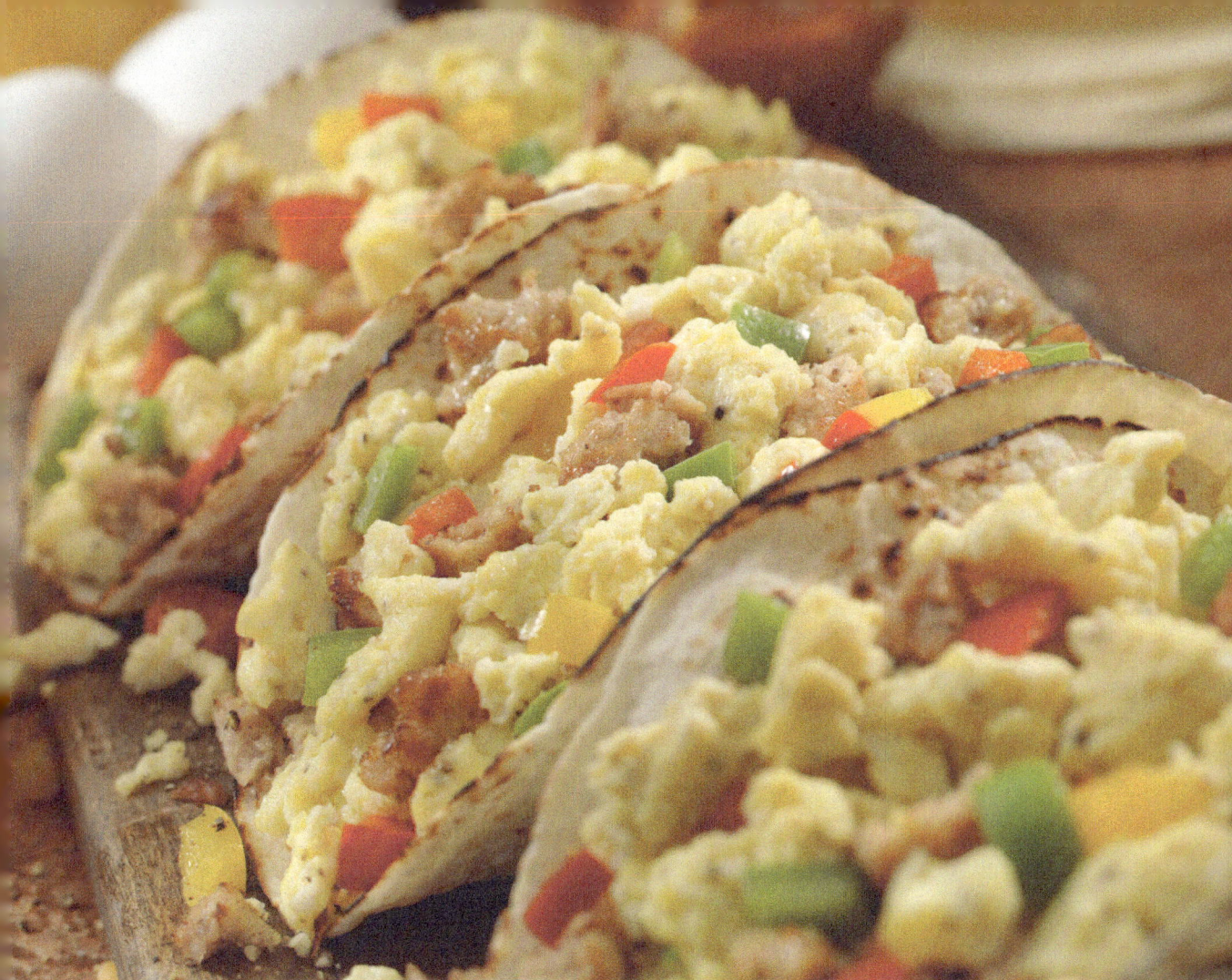

CHAPTER THREE: BREAKFAST

BANANA BREAD OVERNIGHT OATS

Ingredients:
- 1/2 cup rolled oats
- 1/2 cup almond milk
- 1 medium banana
- 1 tbsp. chia seeds
- 1 tsp. vanilla extract
- 1/4 tsp. ground cinnamon

Instructions:
1. In a jar or container with a lid, mix together rolled oats, almond milk, banana, chia seeds, vanilla extract, and ground cinnamon.
2. Stir well and place in the fridge overnight.
3. In the morning, give it a good stir and enjoy cold or heated up!

Serving size: 1 cup
Calories: 290

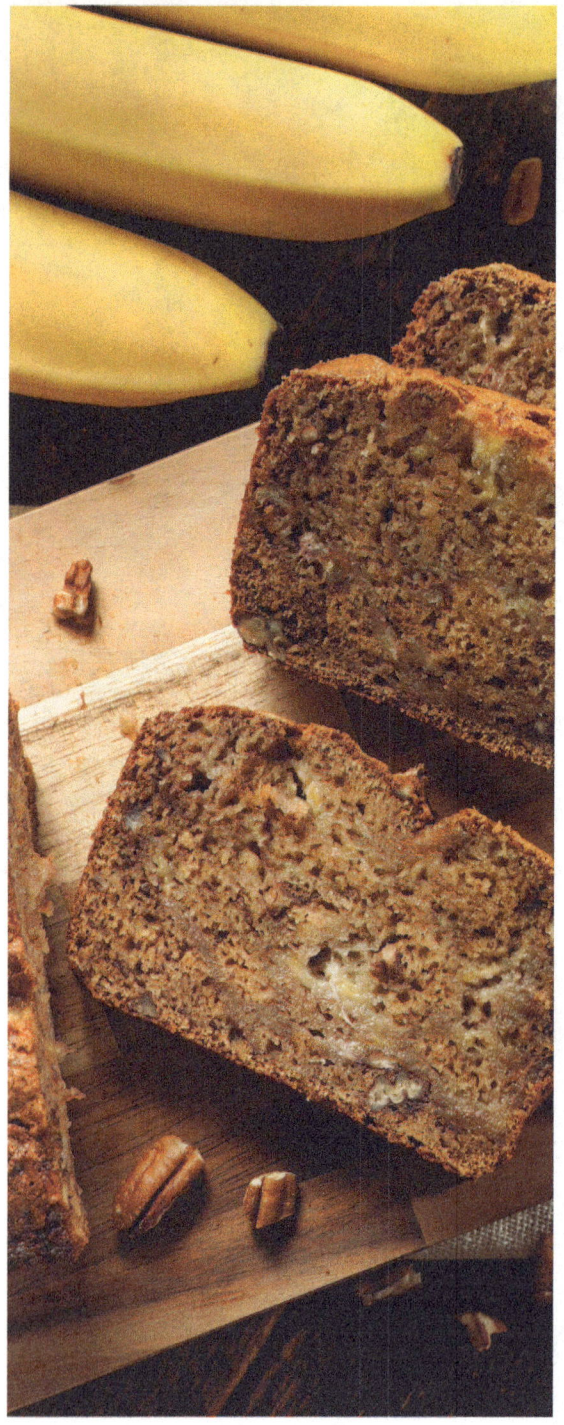

BLUEBERRY ALMOND PANCAKES

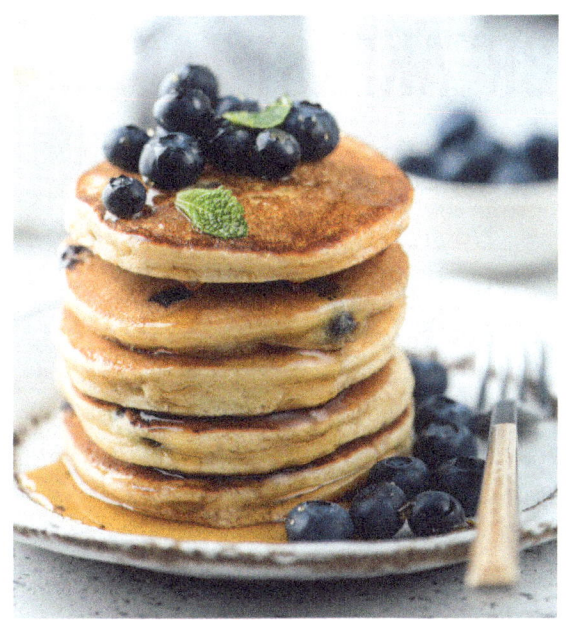

Ingredients:
- 1 cup almond flour
- 1/4 tsp. baking soda
- 1/8 tsp. Salt
- 2 tbsp. Honey
- 1 egg
- 1/4 cup almond milk
- 1 tsp. vanilla extract
- 1/2 cup blueberries

Instructions:
1. In a large bowl, mix together almond flour, baking soda and salt.
2. In a separate bowl, whisk together honey, egg, almond milk and vanilla extract.
3. Pour wet ingredients into the dry ingredients and mix until well combined.
4. Fold in blueberries. Heat a griddle or skillet over medium heat and spray with cooking spray.
5. Scoop 1/4 cup batter onto the griddle for each pancake.
6. Cook for 2-3 minutes per side or until golden brown.
7. Serve with syrup or your favorite toppings!

Serving size: 3 pancakes
Calories: 470

BREAKFAST TACOS

Ingredients:
- 6 eggs
- 1/4 cup milk
- 1/4 tsp. chili powder
- 1/4 tsp. ground cumin
- 1/4 tsp. Salt
- 1 tbsp. olive oil
- 1/2 cup shredded cheddar cheese
- 6 small soft tacos shells
- salsa or hot sauce (optional).

Instructions:
1. In a large bowl, whisk together eggs, milk, chili powder, cumin and salt.
2. Heat a large skillet over medium heat and add olive oil.
3. Pour in the egg mixture and cook until scrambled.
4. Stir in shredded cheese.
5. Spoon into taco shells and enjoy with salsa or hot sauce if desired!

Serving size: 2 tacos
Calories: 350

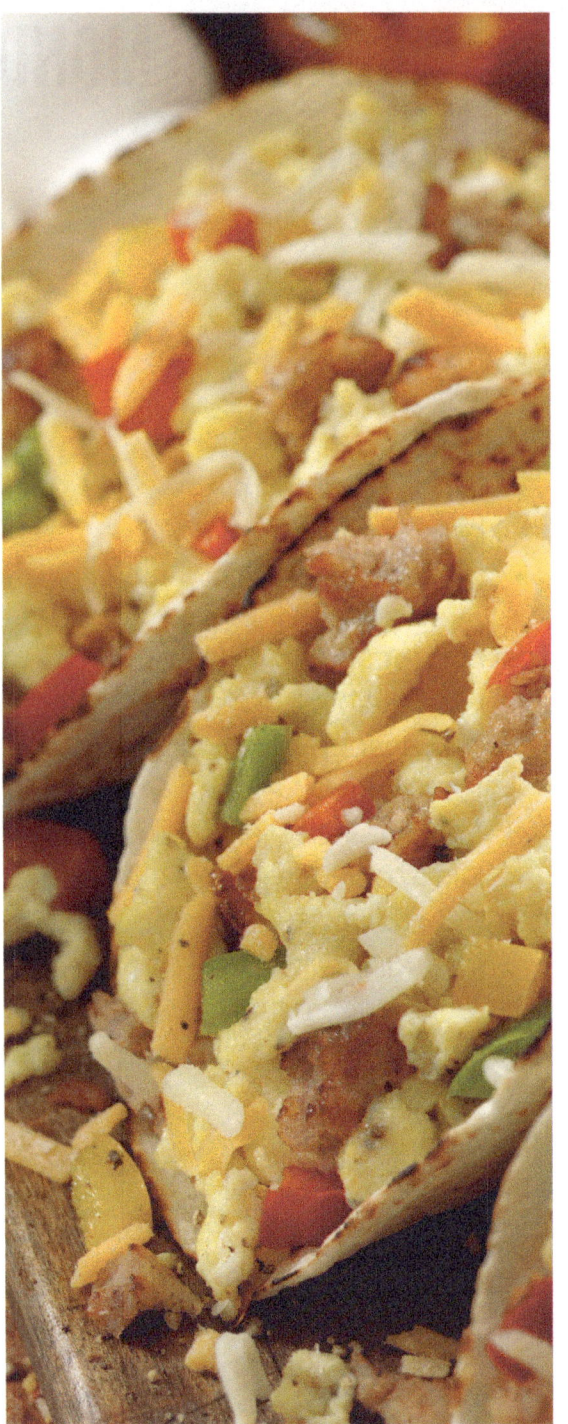

CINNAMON ROLL BAKED OATMEAL

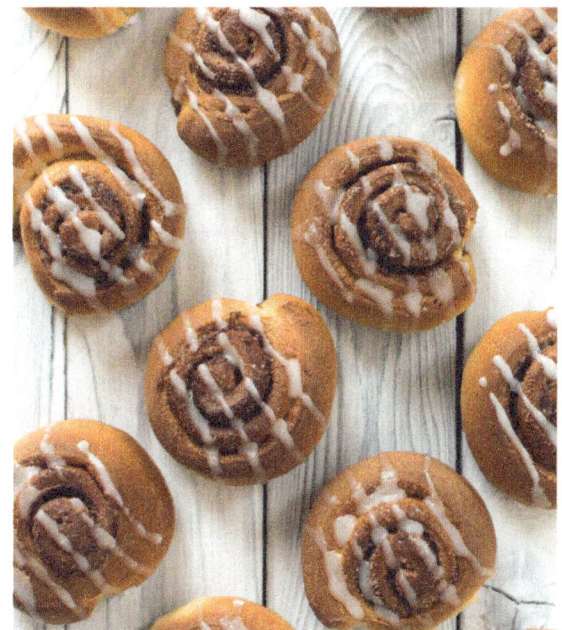

Ingredients:
- 1 cup rolled oats
- 1 tsp. baking powder
- 1/2 tsp. ground cinnamon
- 1/4 tsp. Salt
- 1 cup almond milk
- 2 eggs
- 1/4 cup maple syrup
- 1 tsp. vanilla extract
- 1/2 cup raisins (optional)

Instructions:
1. Preheat oven to 375 degrees F.
2. Mix together rolled oats, baking powder, cinnamon and salt in a large bowl.
3. In a separate bowl whisk together almond milk, eggs, maple syrup and vanilla extract.
4. Pour wet ingredients into the dry ingredients and mix until well combined.
5. Stir in raisins if desired.
6. Pour mixture into an 8x8 inch baking dish sprayed with cooking spray.
7. Bake for 25-30 minutes or until golden brown.
8. Serve with additional maple syrup if desired.

Serving size: 1/2 cup
Calories: 210

PEACH AND ARUGULA SALAD

Ingredients:
- 2 peaches
- 1/4 cup balsamic vinegar
- 2 tbsp. olive oil
- 1/8 tsp salt
- 1/8 tsp. Pepper
- 4 cups arugula
- 1/4 cup crumbled feta cheese

Instructions:
1. Cut the peaches into bite-sized pieces and add to a large bowl.
2. Add balsamic vinegar, olive oil, salt and pepper to the bowl and mix together until well combined.
3. Add arugula and feta cheese to the bowl and mix together until well mixed.
4. Serve immediately!

Serving size: 1 cup
Calories: 190

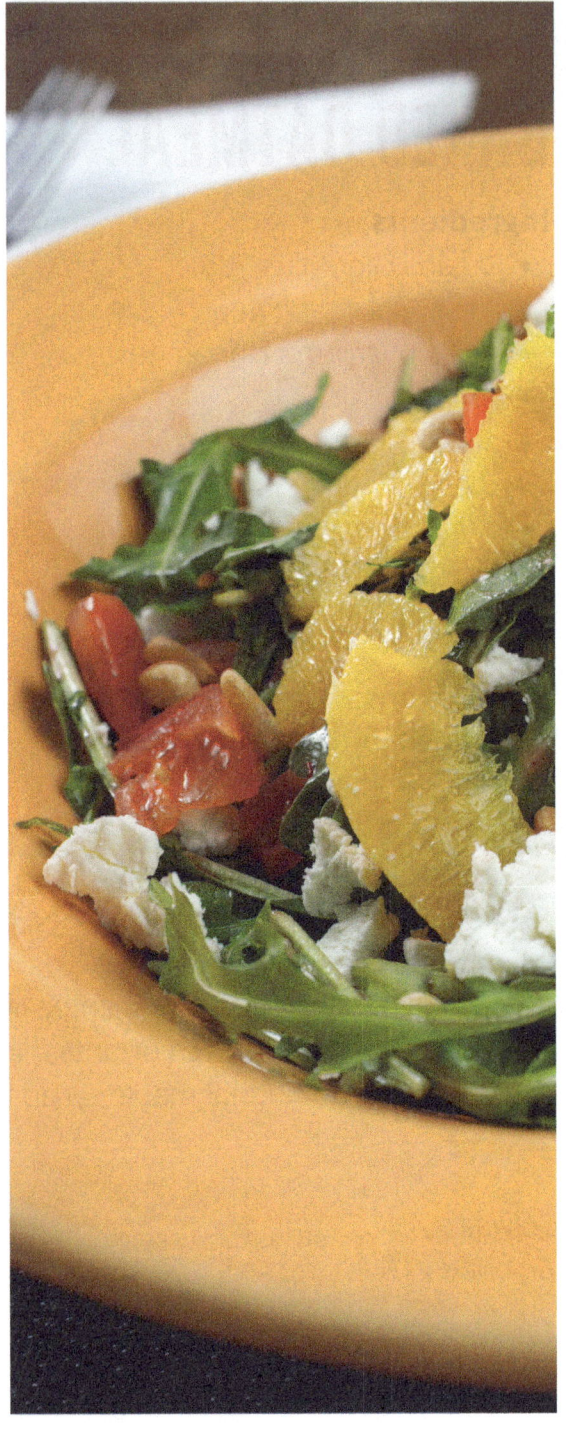

BANANA OATMEAL

Ingredients:
- 1/2 cup rolled oats
- 1 cup water
- 1 banana
- 1 tbsp. Honey
- 1/4 tsp. ground cinnamon

Instructions:
1. Bring the oats and water to a boil in a pot on the stove.
2. Reduce to a simmer and cook for about 5 minutes until the oats are cooked through.
3. Remove from heat and stir in the banana, honey and cinnamon.
4. Enjoy!

Serving size: 1 bowl
Calories: 300

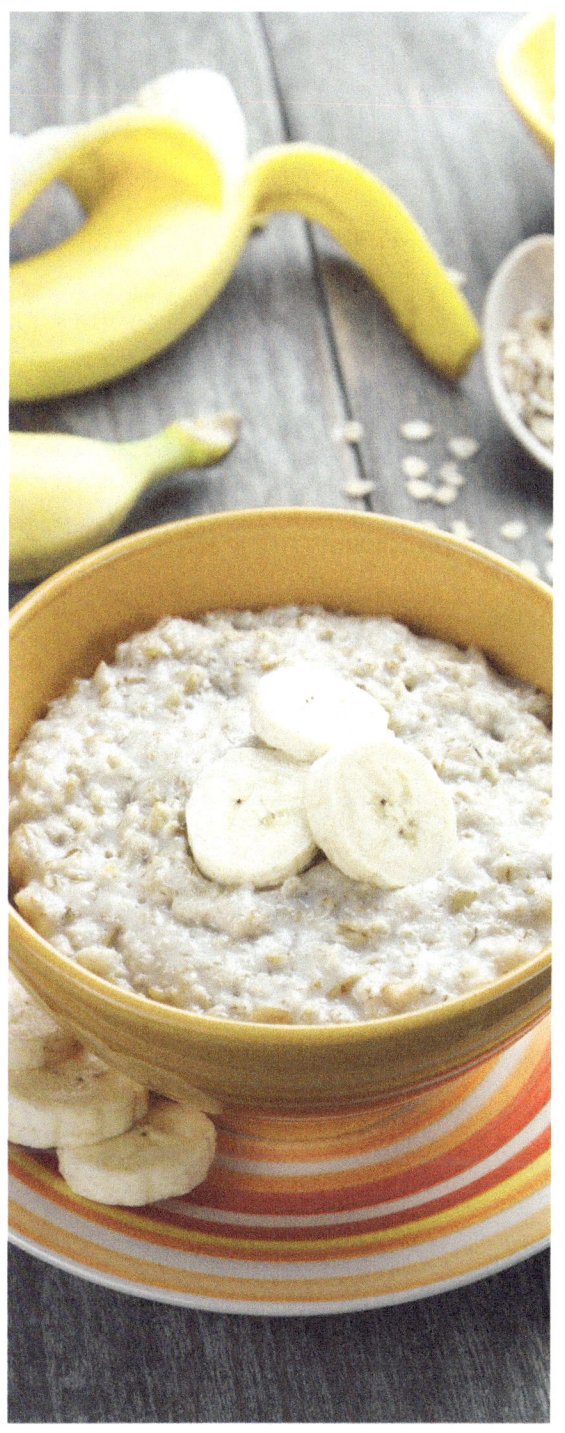

BLUEBERRY MUFFINS

Ingredients:
- 1 cup gluten-free flour
- 1 tsp. baking powder
- 1/4 tsp. salt
- 6 tbsp. butter, softened
- 3/4 cup sugar
- 2 eggs
- 1 tsp. vanilla extract
- 1/2 cup milk
- 1 cup blueberries

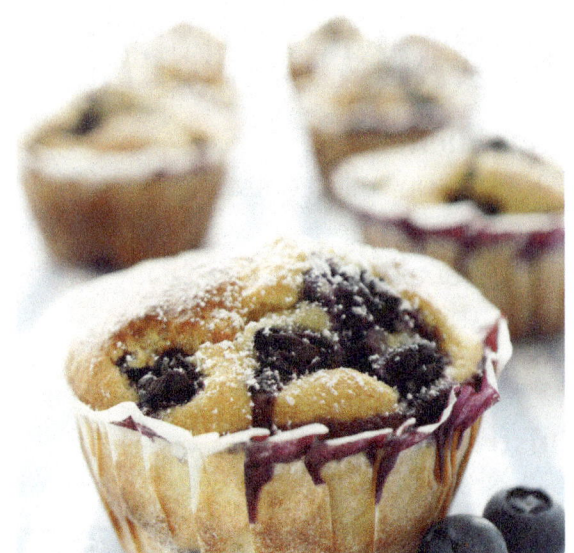

Instructions:
1. Preheat oven to 350 degrees Fahrenheit.
2. In a bowl, whisk together flour, baking powder and salt.
3. In a separate bowl, cream together the butter and sugar until light and fluffy.
4. Beat in the eggs, one at a time, then stir in the vanilla extract.
5. Add the dry ingredients to the wet ingredients in three batches, alternating with the milk.
6. Stir in the blueberries.
7. Divide batter evenly among 12 muffin cups.
8. Bake for about 20 minutes until a toothpick inserted into the center of a muffin comes out clean.

Serving size: 1 muffin
Calories: 250

CHOCOLATE CHIP PANCAKES

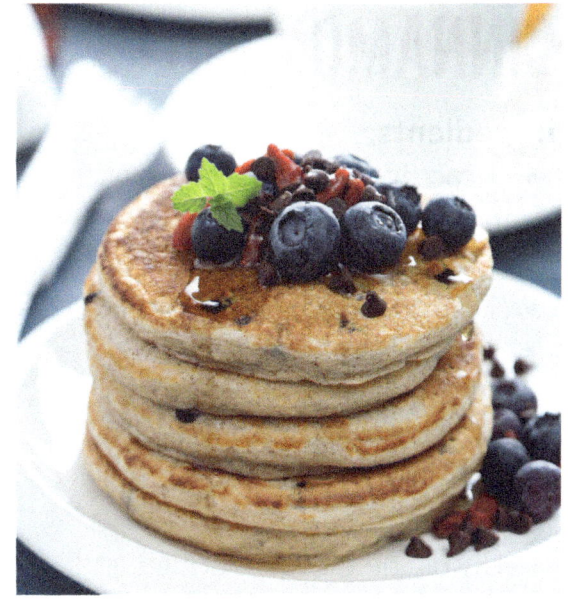

Ingredients:
- 1 cup gluten-free flour
- 1 tsp. baking powder
- 1/4 tsp. Salt
- 2 tbsp. Sugar
- 1 egg
- 1 cup milk
- 2 tbsp. Butter, melted
- 1/2 cup chocolate chips

Instructions:
1. In a bowl, whisk together flour, baking powder and salt.
2. In a separate bowl, whisk together sugar and egg until well combined. '
3. Stir in the milk and melted butter.
4. Add the dry ingredients to the wet ingredients and mix until just combined.
5. Stir in the chocolate chips.
6. Heat a griddle or frying pan over medium heat and grease with butter or cooking spray.
7. Scoop 1/4 cup batter onto the griddle for each pancake.
8. Cook for about 2 minutes per side until golden brown.
9. Serve with syrup or your favorite toppings and enjoy!

Serving size: 3 pancakes
Calories: 400

CINNAMON ROLLS

Ingredients:
- 1 can (8 oz) refrigerated crescent rolls
- 1/4 cup sugar
- 1 tsp. ground cinnamon
- 2 tbsp. butter, melted

Instructions:
1. Preheat oven to 375 degrees Fahrenheit.
2. Unroll the crescent dough and separate into 8 triangles.
3. In a small bowl, mix together sugar and cinnamon.
4. Brush the melted butter on each triangle, then sprinkle with the sugar mixture.
5. Roll up each triangle from the wide end to the narrow end.
6. Place on a baking sheet lined with parchment paper, seam side down.
7. Bake for about 10-12 minutes until golden brown.
8. Serve with icing or your favorite toppings and enjoy!

Serving size: 2 rolls
Calories: 400

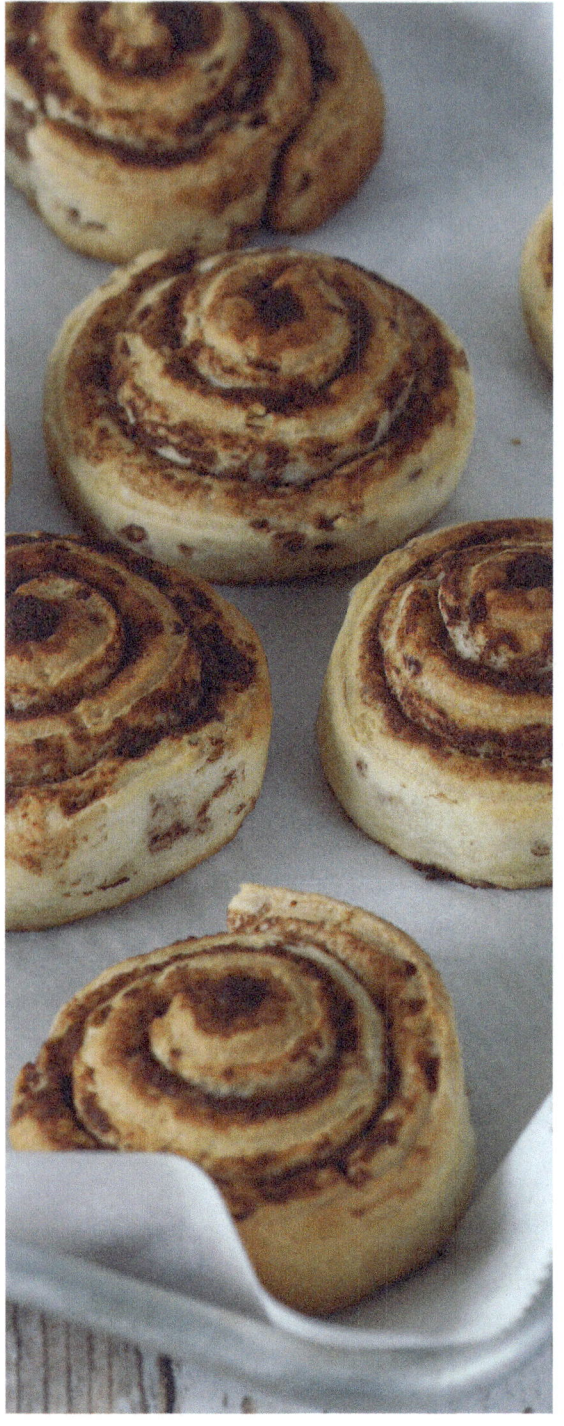

EGG BREAKFAST SANDWICH

Ingredients:
- 2 slices of gluten-free bread
- 2 eggs, cooked to your preference
- 1 slice of cheese, optional

Instructions:
1. Toast the bread.
2. Add the eggs and cheese, if using.
3. Enjoy!

Serving size: 1 sandwich
Calories: 300

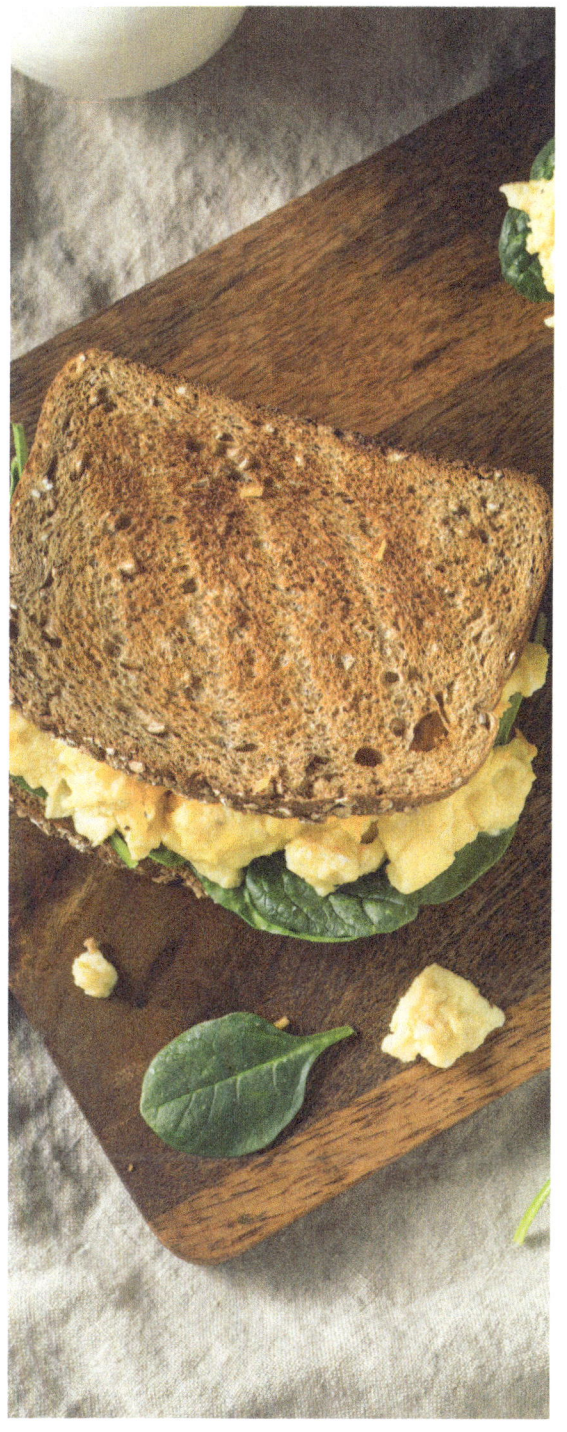

FRUIT SALAD

Ingredients:
- 1/2 cup blueberries
- 1/2 cup raspberries
- 1/2 cup strawberries
- 1/2 banana
- 1 tbsp. Honey

Instructions:
1. Wash and chop the fruit.
2. Add to a bowl with the honey and mix together until well combined.
3. Enjoy!

Serving size: 1 cup
Calories: 100

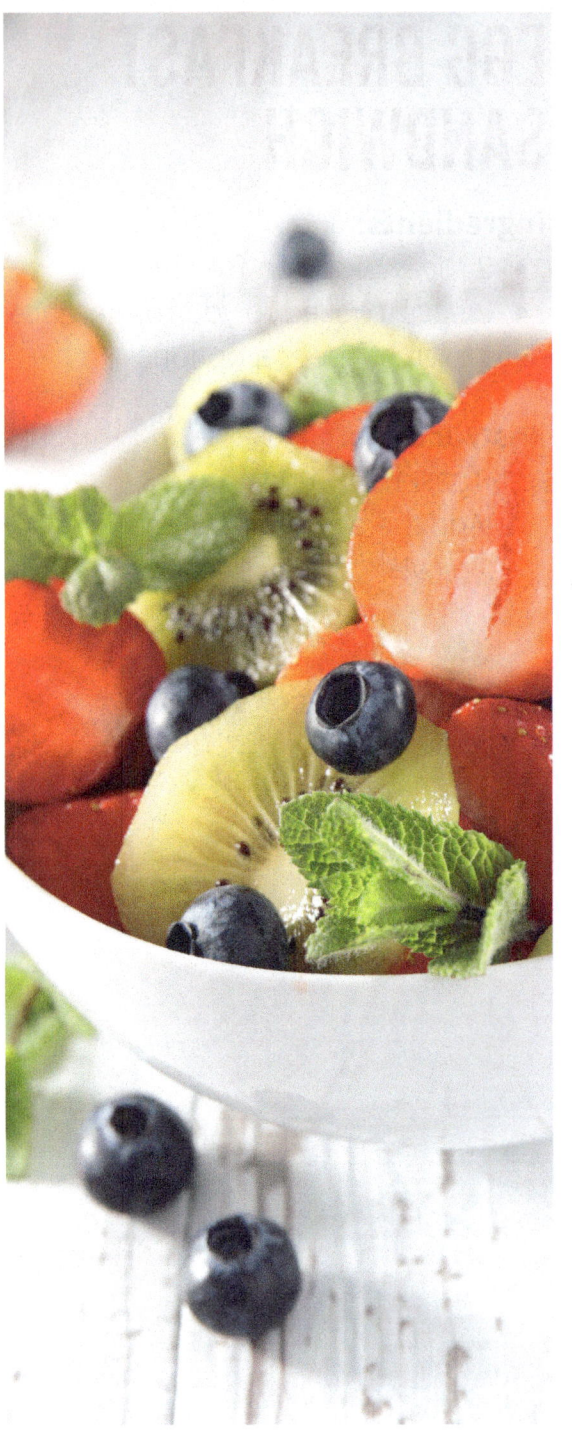

GREEN SMOOTHIE

Ingredients:
- 1 cup spinach
- 1/2 banana
- 1/2 cup almond milk
- 1/2 cup pineapple chunks
- 1 tbsp. chia seeds

Instructions:
1. Add all ingredients to a blender and blend until smooth.
2. Enjoy!

Serving size: 1 cup
Calories: 200

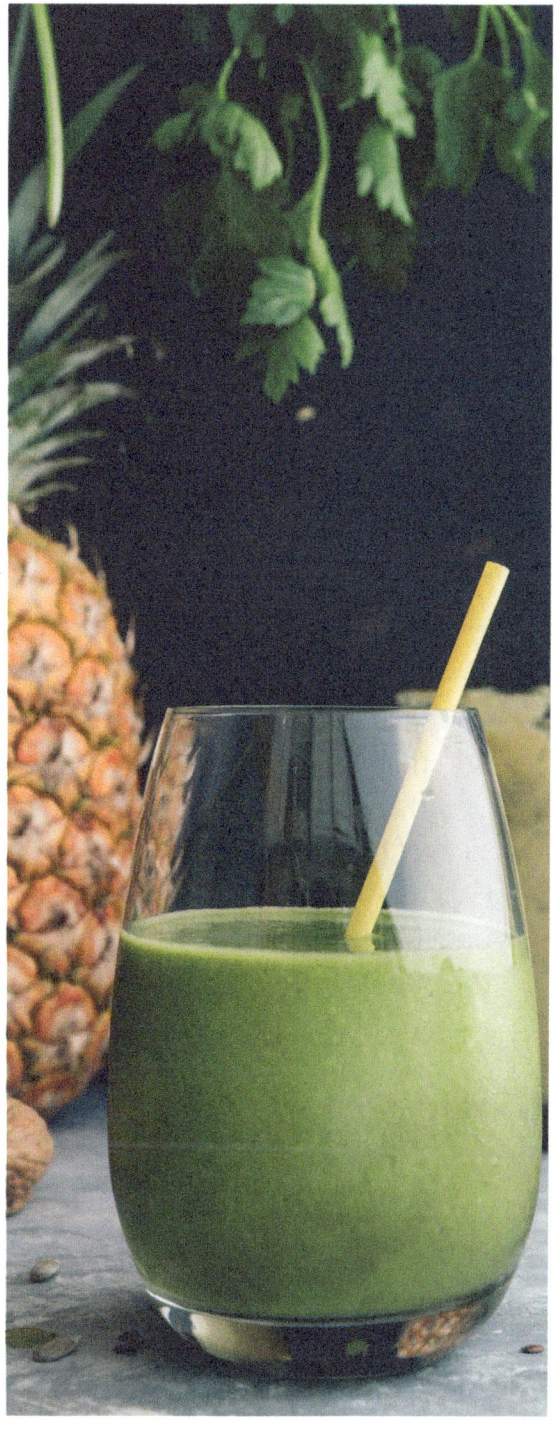

GRILLED CHEESE SANDWICH

Ingredients:
- 2 slices of gluten-free bread
- 2 tbsp. Butter
- 2 slices of cheese

Instructions:
1. Preheat a griddle or frying pan over medium heat.
2. Butter one side of each slice of bread.
3. Place the bread, butter side down, on the griddle or pan.
4. Add the cheese to each slice of bread and then top with the other slice of bread, butter side up.
5. Grill for about 2 minutes per side until the bread is golden brown and the cheese is melted.

Serving size: 1 sandwich
Calories: 400

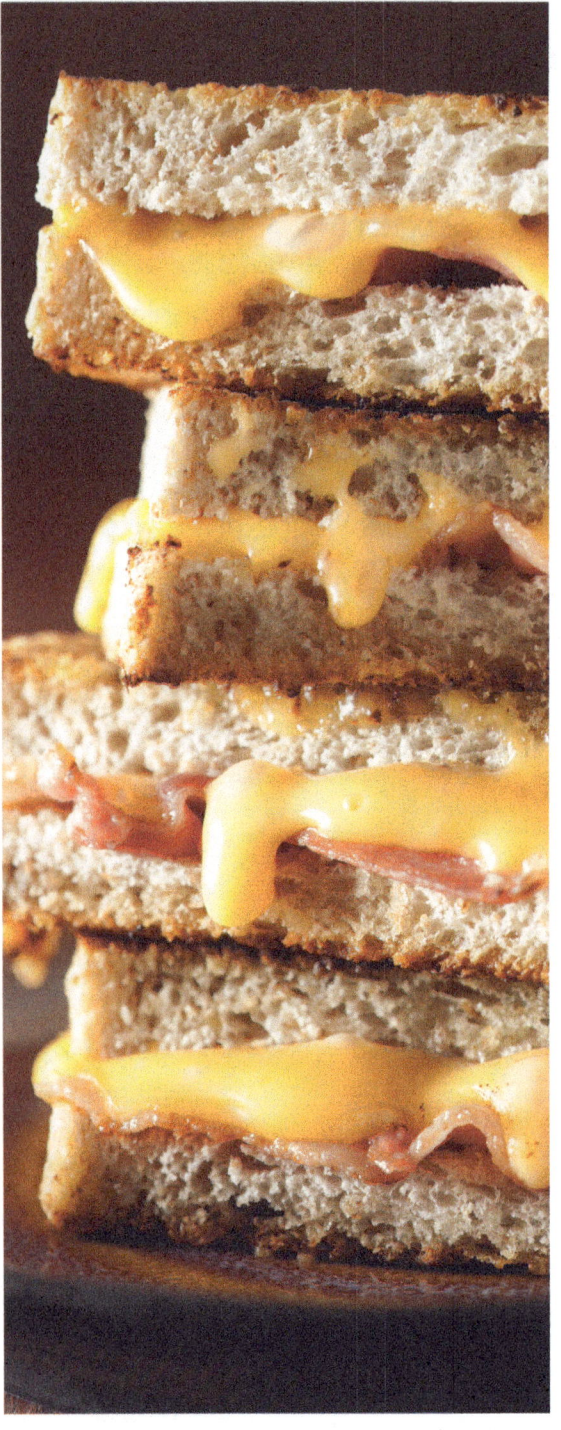

QUICHE

Ingredients:
- 1/2 recipe of gluten-free pie crust
- 1/4 onion, diced
- 3 eggs, beaten
- 1/2 cup milk
- 1/4 tsp. Salt
- 1/4 tsp. black pepper
- 1 cup shredded cheese

Instructions:
1. Preheat oven to 375 degrees Fahrenheit.
2. In a small skillet, cook the onions until they are softened.
3. In a large bowl, whisk together the eggs and milk.
4. Add the salt and pepper and mix well.
5. Stir in the onions and cheese.
6. Pour the mixture into the prepared pie crust.
7. Bake for about 30 minutes or until the quiche is set and golden brown.

Serving size: 1 slice
Calories: 400

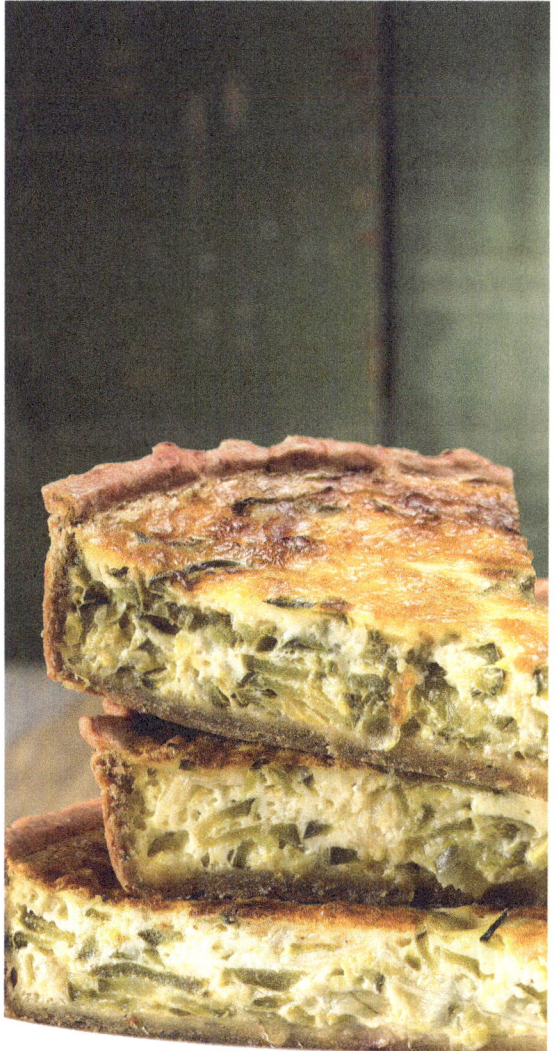

TOMATO SOUP

Ingredients:
- 2 cans (14 oz) diced tomatoes
- 2 cups chicken or vegetable broth
- 1 onion, diced
- 1 carrot, diced
- 1 celery stalk, diced
- 1/4 tsp. Salt
- 1/4 tsp. black pepper

Instructions:
1. Add all ingredients to a large pot or Dutch oven and stir together.
2. Bring the soup to a simmer over medium heat and cook for about 10 minutes until the vegetables are softened.
3. Use an immersion blender to puree the soup until it is smooth.
4. Alternatively, you can transfer the soup in batches to a regular blender and blend until smooth.

Serving size: 1 cup
Calories: 100

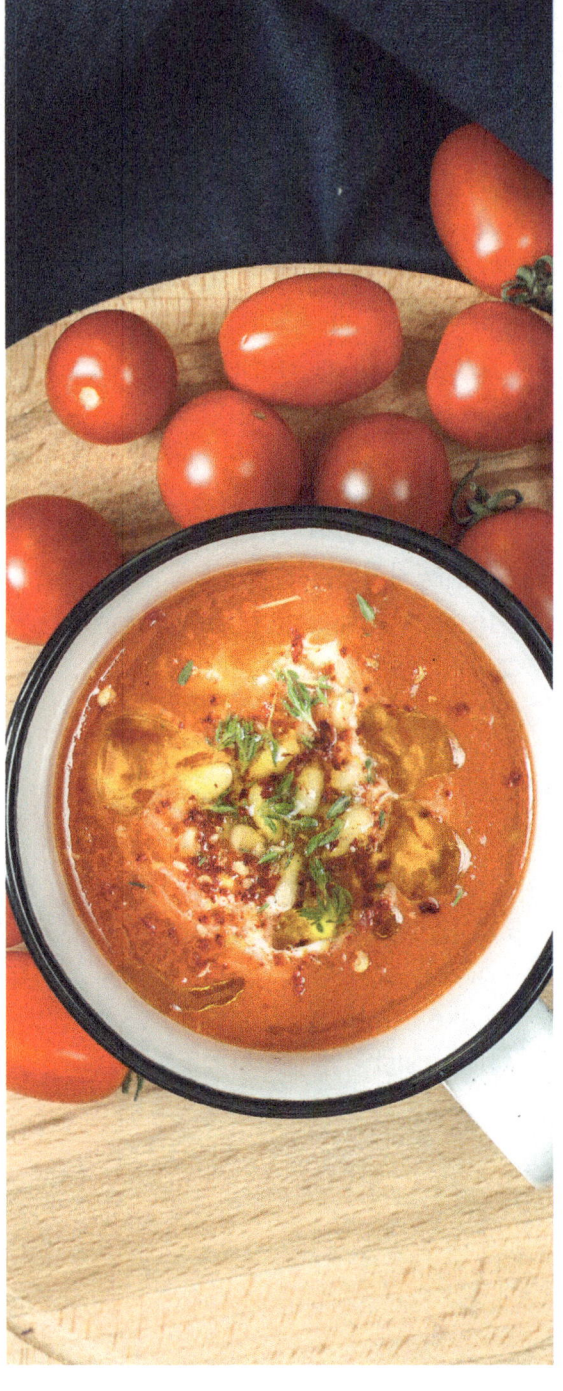

OMELET WITH VEGETABLES

Ingredients:
- 3 eggs
- 1/4 cup diced onion
- 1/4 cup diced bell pepper
- 1/4 cup diced mushrooms
- 1 tablespoon olive oil
- salt and pepper to taste.

Instructions:
1. In a large skillet over medium heat, sauté onions, bell peppers, and mushrooms in olive oil until tender.
2. Add salt and pepper to taste.
3. Whisk together eggs and pour into the pan.
4. Cook until the eggs are firm and the edges are golden brown.

Serving size: 1 omelet
Calories: approximately 300

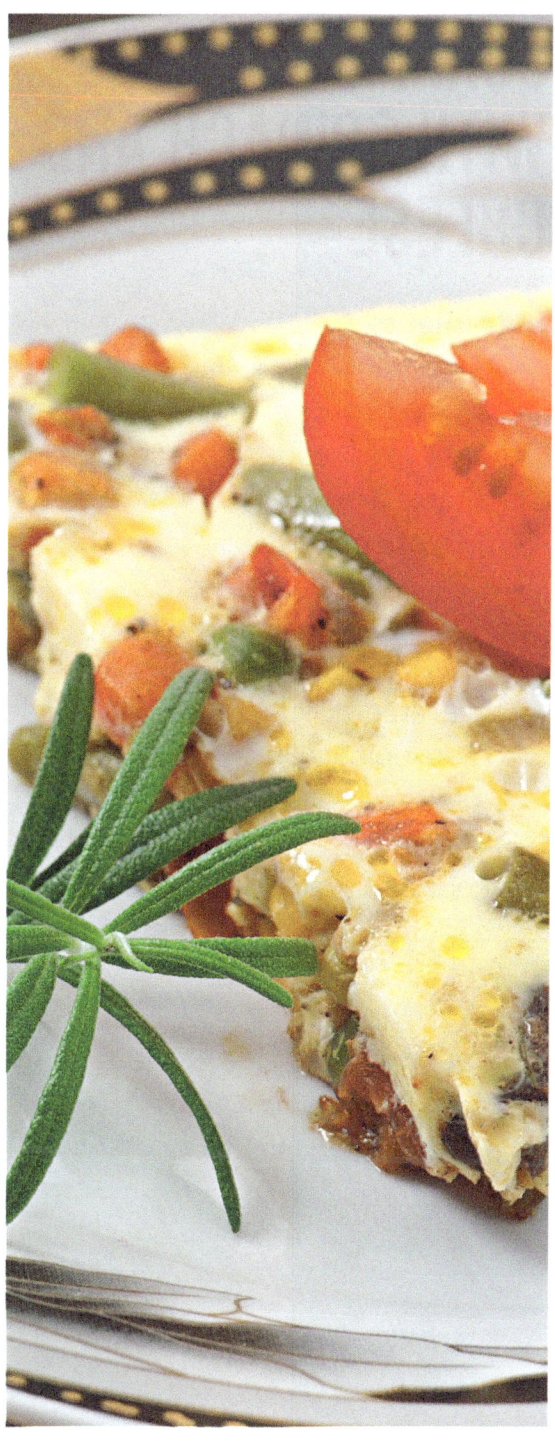

SCRAMBLED EGGS WITH SPINACH AND CHEESE

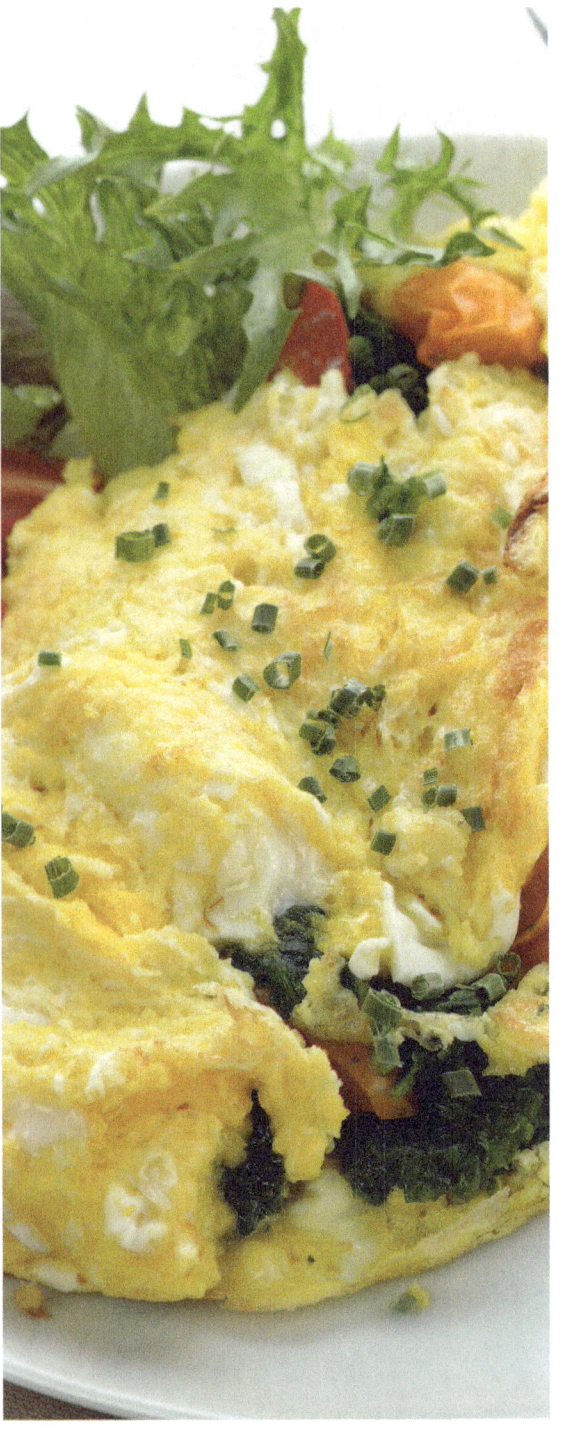

Ingredients:
- 3 eggs
- 1/2 cup chopped spinach
- 1/4 cup shredded cheese
- 1 tablespoon milk
- 1 teaspoon olive oil
- salt and pepper to taste.

Instructions:
1. In a large skillet over medium heat, sauté spinach in olive oil until wilted.
2. Add salt and pepper to taste.
3. Whisk together eggs, milk, and cheese
4. Pour into the pan and cook until the eggs are firm and the edges are golden brown.

Serving size: 1 serving
Calories: approximately 300

SAUSAGE AND EGG BREAKFAST BURRITO

Ingredients:
- 1 gluten-free tortilla
- 1/4 cup cooked sausage
- 1 egg, scrambled
- 1 tablespoon shredded cheese
- salsa, optional.

Instructions:
1. Preheat a skillet over medium heat.
2. Add the sausage to the pan and cook until browned.
3. Add the scrambled egg and cheese to the tortilla, then top with salsa if desired.
4. Roll up the burrito and serve warm.
5. Enjoy!

Serving size: 1 burrito
Calories: 400-500

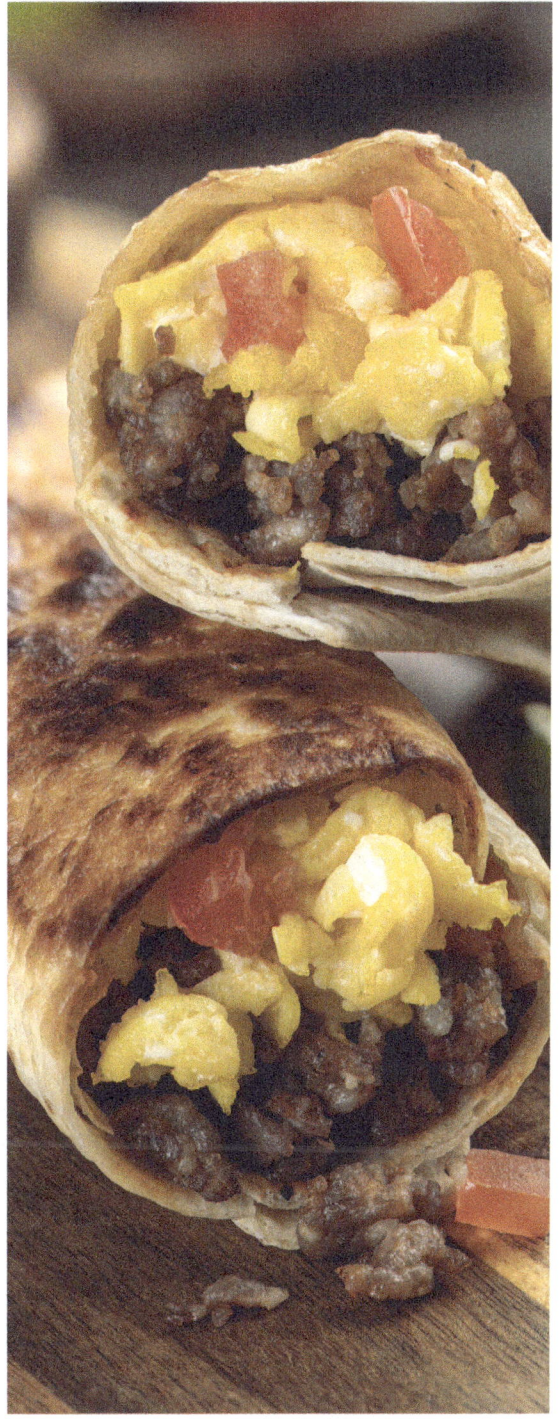

BANANA PANCAKES

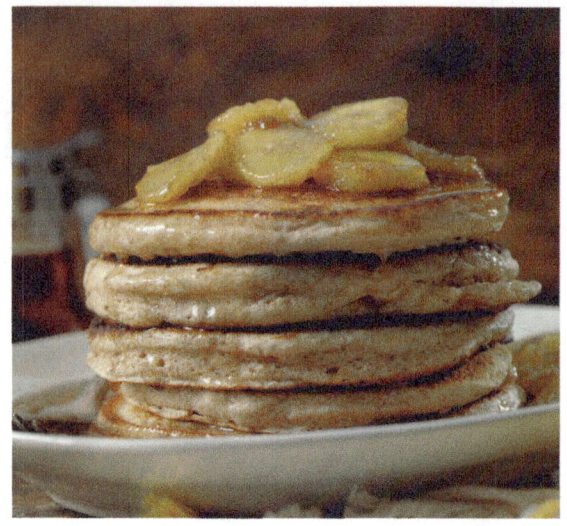

Ingredients:
- 1 cup gluten-free flour
- 2 tablespoons sugar
- 2 teaspoons baking powder
- 1/4 teaspoon salt
- 1 egg, beaten
- 1 cup milk
- 2 tablespoons melted butter
- 1 banana, mashed.

Instructions:
1. In a large bowl, whisk together the flour, sugar, baking powder, and salt. In another bowl, whisk together the egg, milk, and melted butter. Stir the wet ingredients into the dry ingredients until just combined. Fold in the mashed banana.
2. Preheat a griddle or frying pan over medium heat. Grease with butter or cooking spray. For each pancake, spoon 1/4 cup of batter onto the griddle. Cook for 1-2 minutes or until bubbles form on the surface of the pancakes and then flip. Cook for an additional minute or until golden brown.
3. Serve with maple syrup and enjoy!

Serving size: 2 pancakes
Calories: 400

QUINOA BREAKFAST BOWL

Ingredients:
- 1/2 cup cooked quinoa
- 1/2 banana, sliced
- 1 tablespoon almond butter
- 1/4 cup chopped almonds
- 1/4 cup dried cranberries.

Instructions:
1. In a bowl, combine cooked quinoa, banana, almond butter, chopped almonds, and dried cranberries.
2. Enjoy as is or warm in the microwave for 1-2 minutes.

Serving size: 1 bowl
Calories: 400

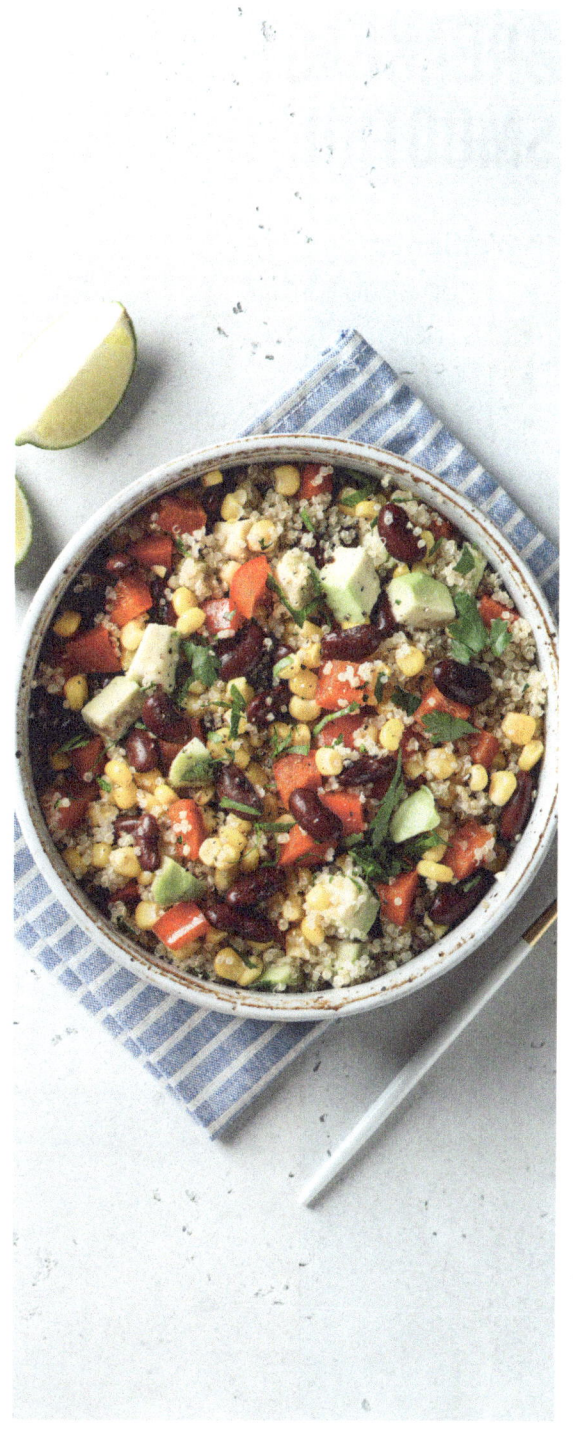

BREAKFAST SMOOTHIE

Ingredients:
- 1 cup almond milk
- 1/2 banana, frozen
- 1/4 cup oats
- 1 tablespoon chia seeds

Instructions:
1. Add all ingredients to a blender and blend until smooth.
2. Enjoy as is or pour into a bowl and top with your favorite fruit, nuts, and/or seeds.
3. Enjoy!

Serving size: 1 smoothie
Calories: approximately 300

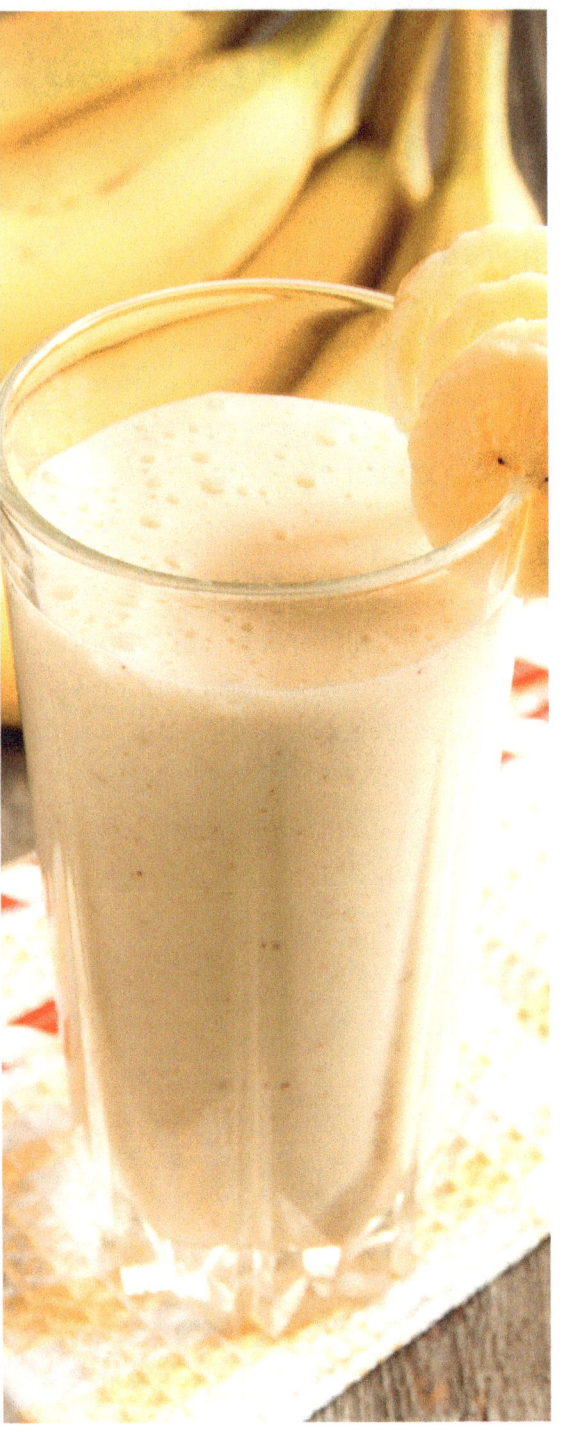

GREEK YOGURT WITH FRUIT AND HONEY

Ingredients:
- 1 cup plain Greek yogurt
- 1/2 cup fresh berries or diced fruit
- 1 tablespoon honey

Instructions:
1. In a bowl, combine Greek yogurt, berries or diced fruit, and honey.
2. Enjoy!

Serving size: 1 serving
Calories: 400

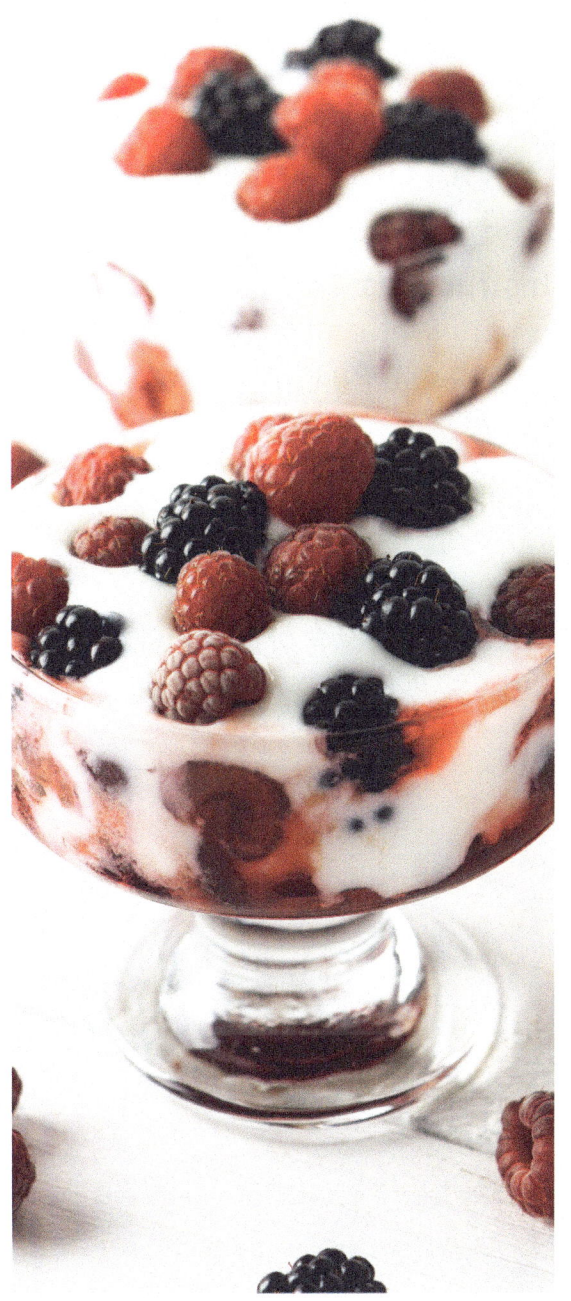

AVOCADO TOAST

Ingredients:
- 1 slice gluten-free bread
- 1/2 avocado, mashed
- 1 hard-boiled egg, sliced
- salt and pepper to taste.

Instructions:
1. Spread the toast with avocado and top with a hard-boiled egg.
2. Season with salt and pepper to taste.
3. Enjoy!

Serving size: 1 slice of toast
Calories: approximately 300

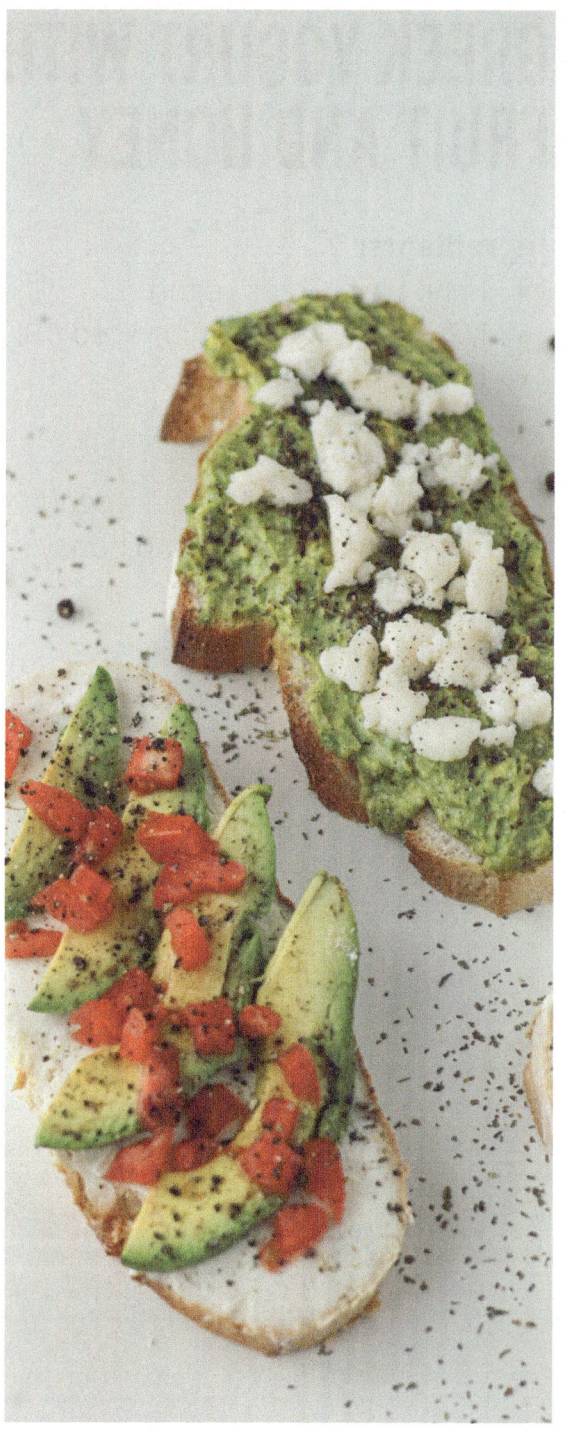

SMOKED SALMON BAGEL

Ingredients:
- 1/2 bagel, toasted
- 1 ounce cream cheese, softened
- 1/4 cup smoked salmon
- 1/4 teaspoon capers, optional.

Instructions:
1. Spread the Bagel with cream cheese.
2. Top with smoked salmon and capers, if desired.
3. Enjoy!

Serving size: 1/2 bagel
Calories: 400-500

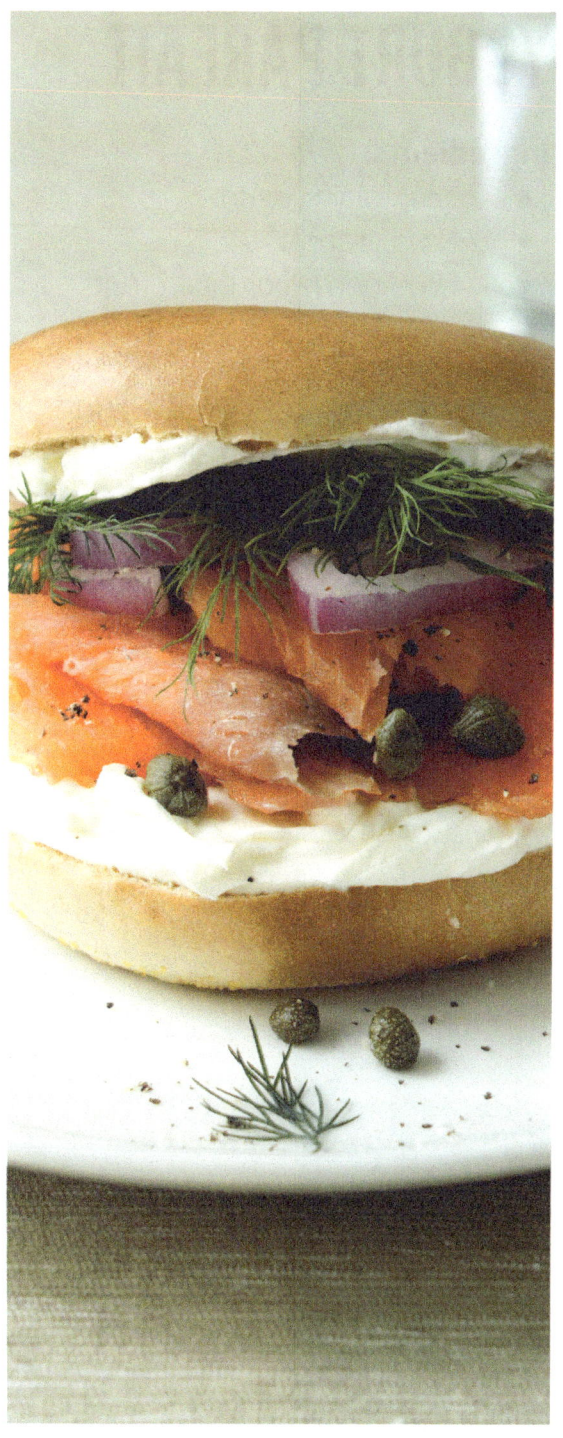

YOGURT PARFAIT

Ingredients:
- 1/2 cup plain yogurt
- 1/4 cup granola
- 1/4 cup berries or diced fruit.

Instructions:
1. In a bowl or glass, layer yogurt, granola, and berries or diced fruit.
2. Enjoy!

Serving size: 1 parfait
Calories: approximately 300

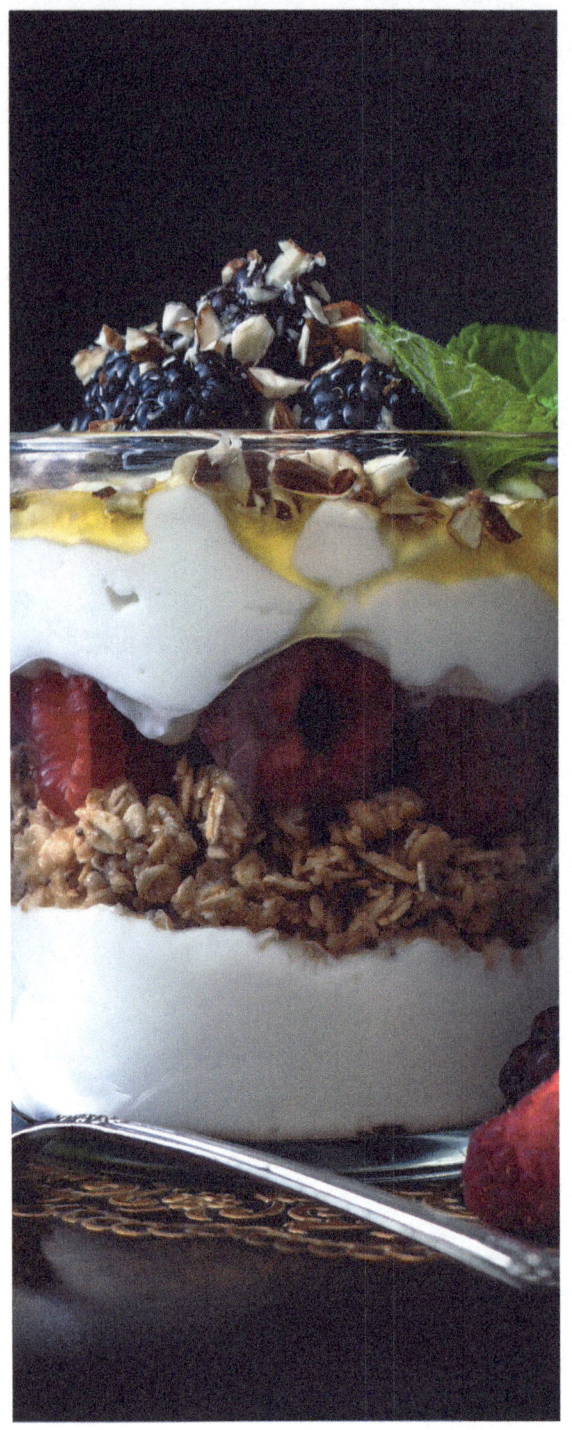

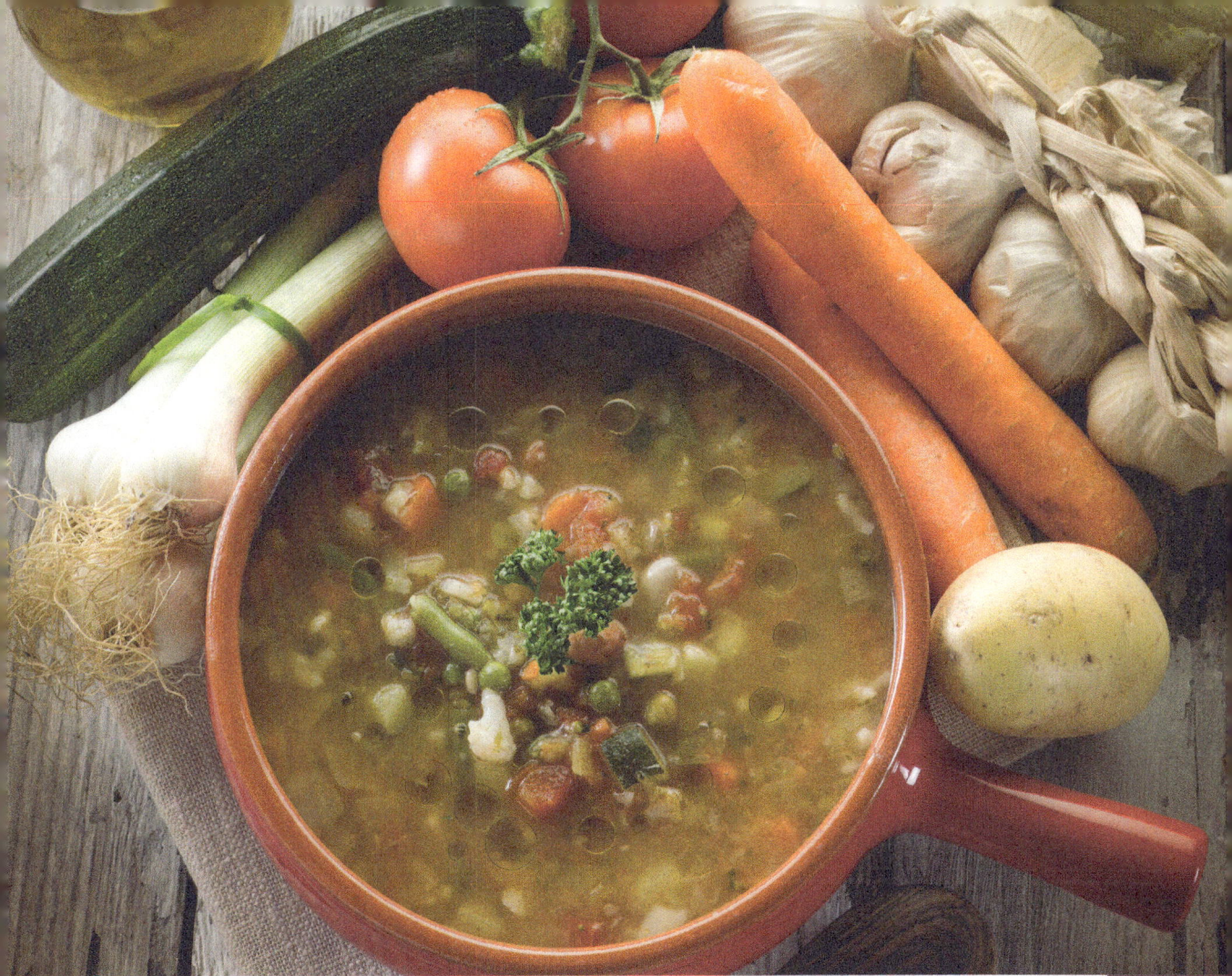

CHAPTER FOUR: LUNCHES

QUINOA VEGGIE BOWL

Ingredients:
- 1 cup cooked quinoa
- 1/2 cup diced tomatoes
- 1/2 cup cooked black beans
- 1/4 cup chopped onion
- 1/4 cup diced avocado
- 1 tbsp. lime juice
- salt and pepper to taste.

Instructions:
1. Add all ingredients to a large bowl and mix together until well combined.
2. Serve as is or with your favorite dressing!

Serving size: 1 cup
Calories: 380

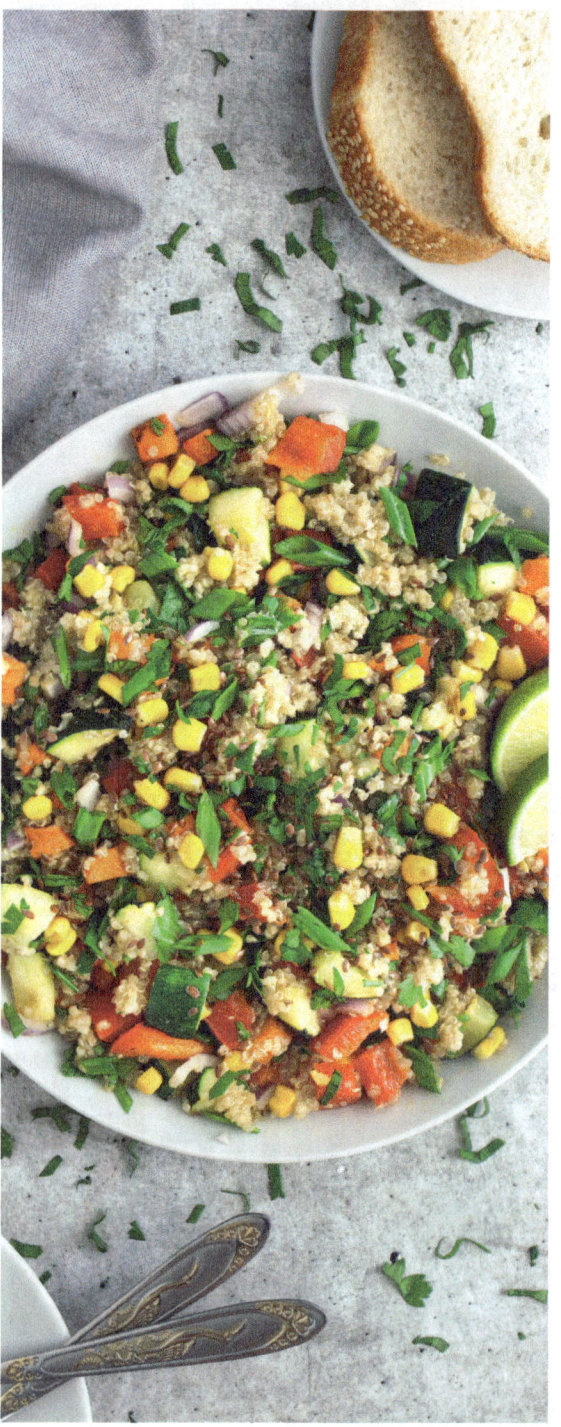

SPICY THAI PEANUT NOODLES

Ingredients:
- 8 oz. rice noodles
- 2 tbsp. peanut butter
- 1 tbsp. soy sauce
- 1 tbsp. Honey
- 1 tbsp. rice vinegar
- 1 tsp. sesame oil
- 1/2 tsp. red pepper flakes
- 1 clove garlic, minced
- 1/4 cup chopped green onions
- 1/4 cup chopped peanuts (optional)

Instructions:
1. Cook rice noodles according to package instructions.
2. In a large bowl whisk together peanut butter, soy sauce, honey, rice vinegar, sesame oil, red pepper flakes and garlic until well combined.
3. Add cooked noodles and green onions to the bowl and mix together until well mixed.
4. Top with chopped peanuts if desired!

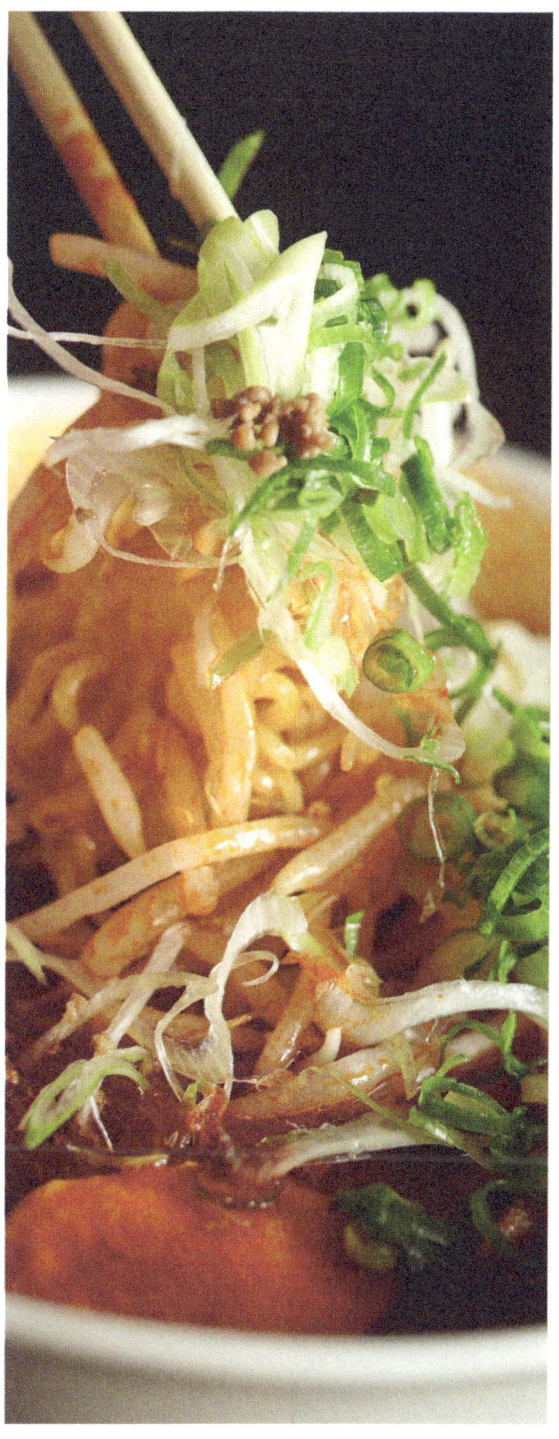

Serving size: 1 cup
Calories: 440

GREEK YOGURT CHICKEN SALAD

Ingredients:
- 2 cups cooked chicken
- 1/2 cup diced celery
- 1/4 cup chopped green onions
- 1/4 cup chopped grapes
- 1/2 cup plain Greek yogurt
- 2 tbsp. Mayonnaise
- 1 tsp. Dijon mustard
- salt and pepper to taste

Instructions:
1. Add all ingredients to a large bowl and mix together until well combined.
2. Serve on a bed of greens or in a sandwich.

Serving size: 1 cup
Calories: 330

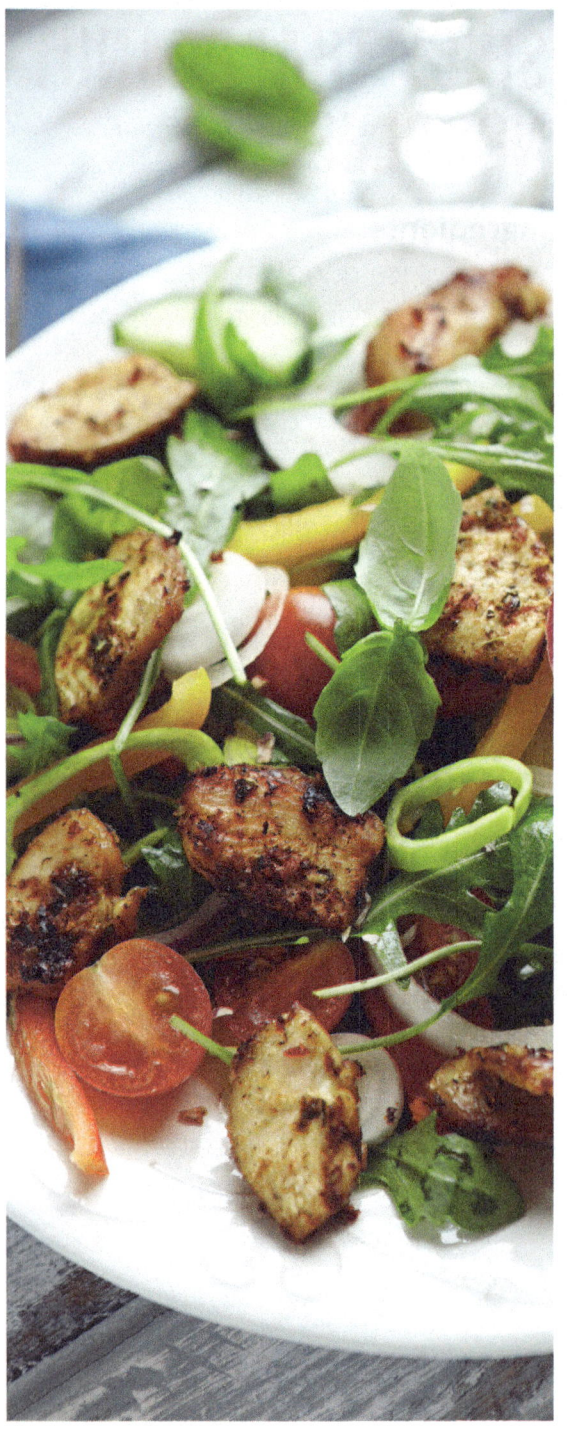

SPICY BLACK BEAN SOUP

Ingredients:
- 1 can black beans
- 2 cups vegetable broth
- 1/2 diced onion
- 1 diced green bell pepper
- 2 cloves minced garlic
- 1 tsp. chili powder
- 1 tsp. ground cumin
- salt and pepper to taste

Instructions:
1. Add all ingredients to a large pot and bring to a boil.
2. Reduce heat and simmer for 10 minutes.
3. Use an immersion blender or regular blender to blend soup until desired consistency is reached.
4. Serve with shredded cheese and sour cream if desired!

Serving size: 1 cup
Calories: 120

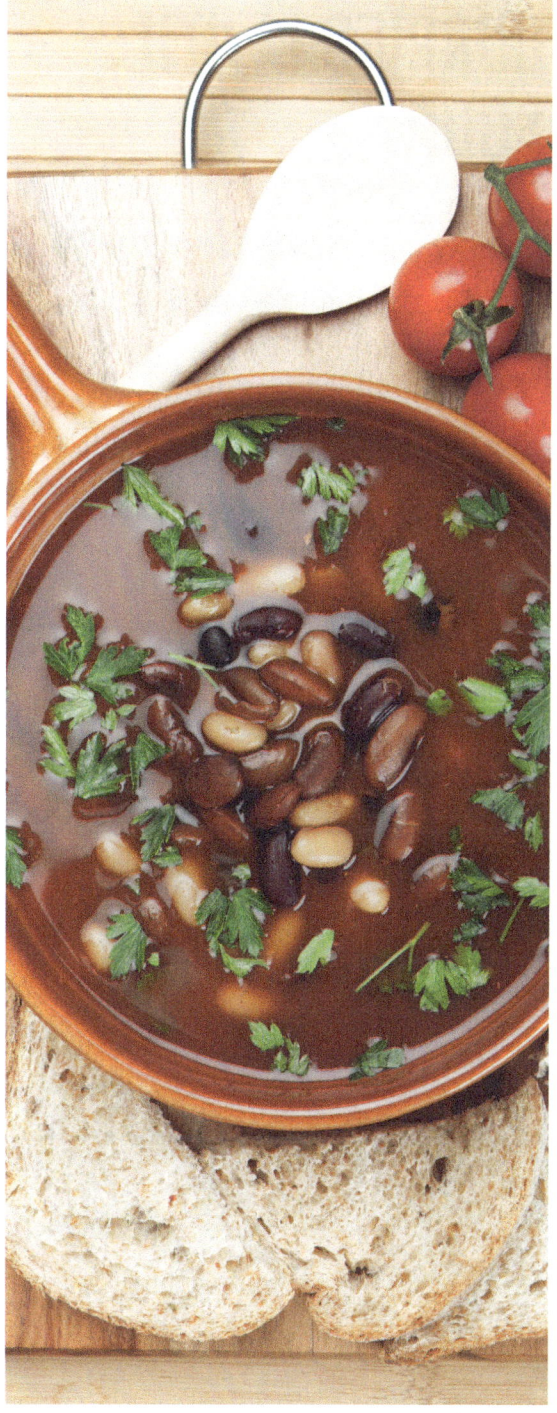

CURRIED LENTIL SOUP

Ingredients:
- 1 cup dried lentils
- 2 cups vegetable broth
- 1/2 diced onion
- 2 cloves minced garlic
- 1 tsp. curry powder
- salt and pepper to taste

Instructions:
1. Add all ingredients to a large pot and bring to a boil.
2. Reduce heat and simmer for 20 minutes or until lentils are cooked through.
3. Use an immersion blender or regular blender to blend soup until desired consistency is reached.
4. Serve with chopped cilantro if desired!

Serving size: 1 cup
Calories: 170

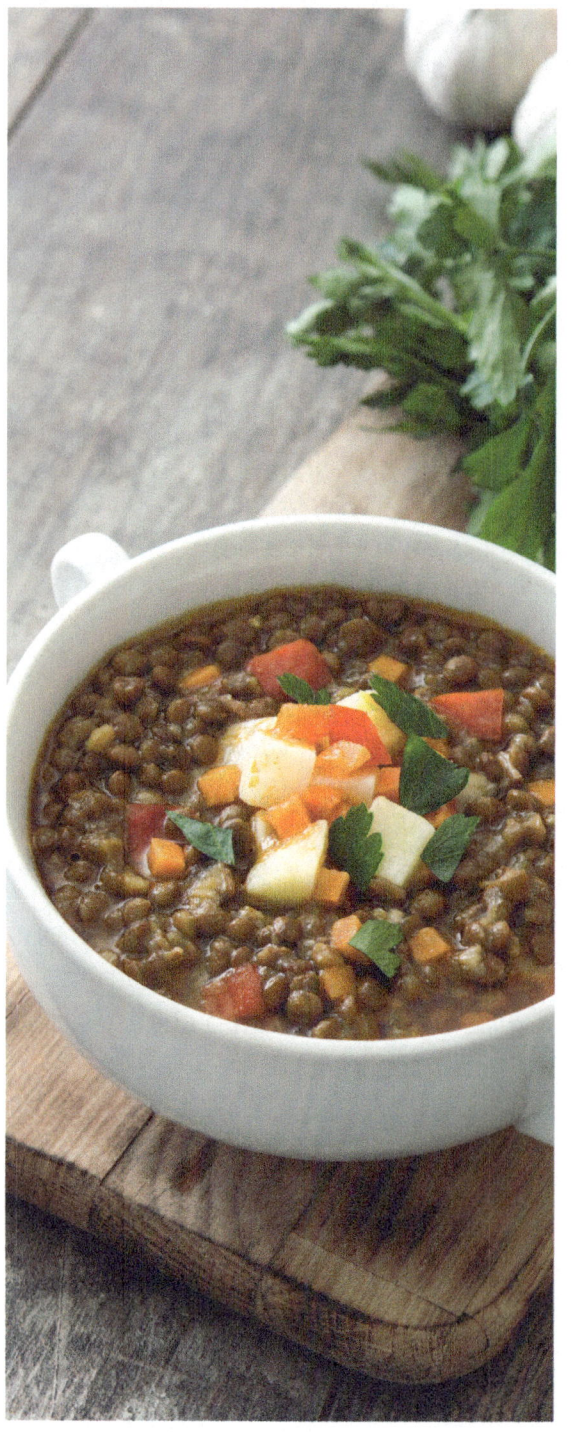

TOMATO BASIL SOUP

Ingredients:
- 2 cans diced tomatoes
- 2 cups vegetable broth
- 1/4 cup chopped onion
- 2 cloves minced garlic
- 1 tbsp. olive oil
- 1 tsp. Sugar
- 1/4 cup chopped fresh basil
- salt and pepper to taste

Instructions:
1. Add all ingredients to a large pot and bring to a boil.
2. Reduce heat and simmer for 10 minutes.
3. Use an immersion blender or regular blender to blend soup until desired consistency is reached.
4. Serve with shredded Parmesan cheese if desired!

Serving size: 1 cup
Calories: 90

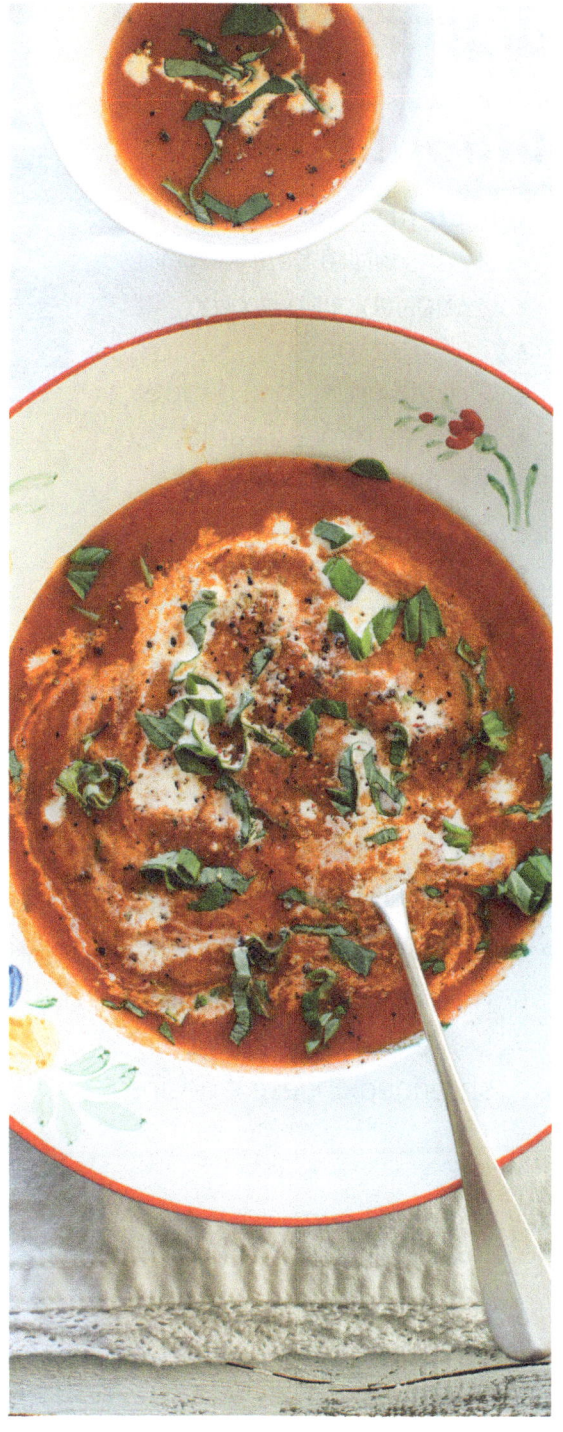

WHITE BEAN CHICKEN CHILI

Ingredients:
- 2 cans white beans
- 2 cups chicken broth
- 1/2 diced onion
- 1 diced green bell pepper
- 2 cloves minced garlic
- 1 tsp. chili powder
- 1 tsp. ground cumin
- 1/4 cup chopped fresh cilantro
- salt and pepper to taste

Instructions:
1. Add all ingredients to a large pot and bring to a boil.
2. Reduce heat and simmer for 10 minutes.
3. Use an immersion blender or regular blender to blend soup until desired consistency is reached.
4. Serve with sour cream and shredded cheese if desired!

Serving size: 1 cup
Calories: 210

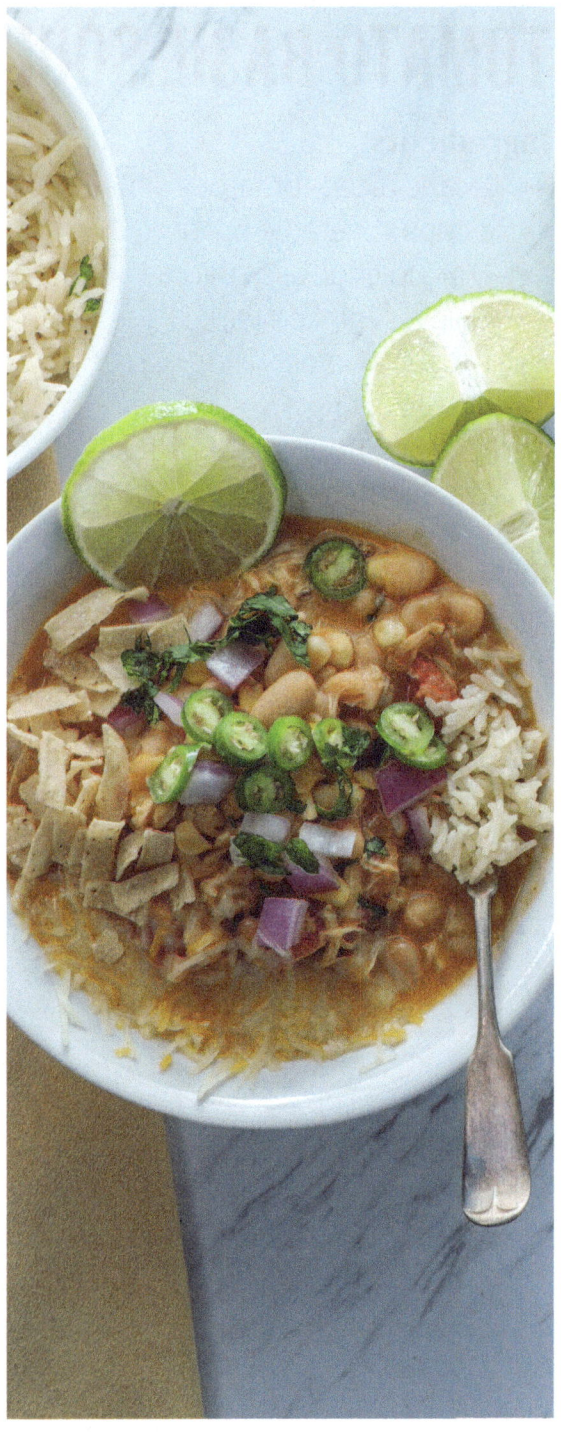

SPICY BLACK BEAN BURGER WITH AVOCADO MAYO AND ROASTED SWEET POTATO WEDGES

Ingredients:
- 1 can black beans, drained and rinsed
- 1/2 cup cooked brown rice
- 1/4 cup diced onion
- 1 egg
- 1 tablespoon chili powder
- 1 teaspoon ground cumin
- 1/4 teaspoon salt
- 1 tablespoon olive oil
- 4 gluten-free hamburger buns
- 1 avocado, diced
- 1/4 cup diced tomatoes
- 1/4 cup organic mayonnaise

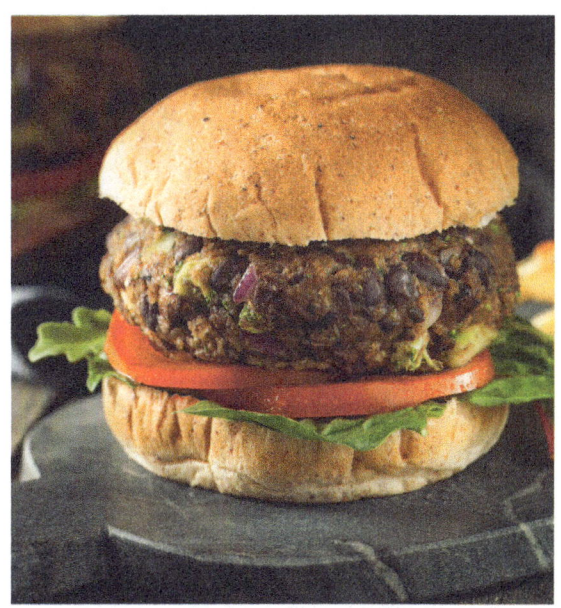

Instructions:
1. In a large bowl, mash the black beans with a fork or potato masher. Mix in the rice, onion, egg, chili powder, cumin, and salt. Divide mixture into four patties.
2. Heat olive oil in a large skillet over medium heat. Add the patties and cook until browned and firm, about five minutes per side.
3. To assemble the burgers, spread avocado mayo on the hamburger buns. Top with a black bean patty, diced tomatoes, and organic mayonnaise.

Serving size: 1 burger
Calories: 590

QUINOA SALAD WITH ROASTED VEGETABLES

Ingredients:
- 1 cup cooked and cooled quinoa
- 1 roasted red pepper, diced
- 1/4 cup crumbled feta cheese
- 1/4 cup chopped fresh parsley
- 1 tablespoon olive oil
- 2 tablespoons freshly squeezed lemon juice
- 1 clove garlic, minced
- salt and pepper to taste

Instructions:
1. In a large bowl, mix together cooked quinoa, roasted red pepper, feta cheese, parsley, olive oil, lemon juice, garlic, salt, and pepper.

Serving size: 1 cup
Calories: 220

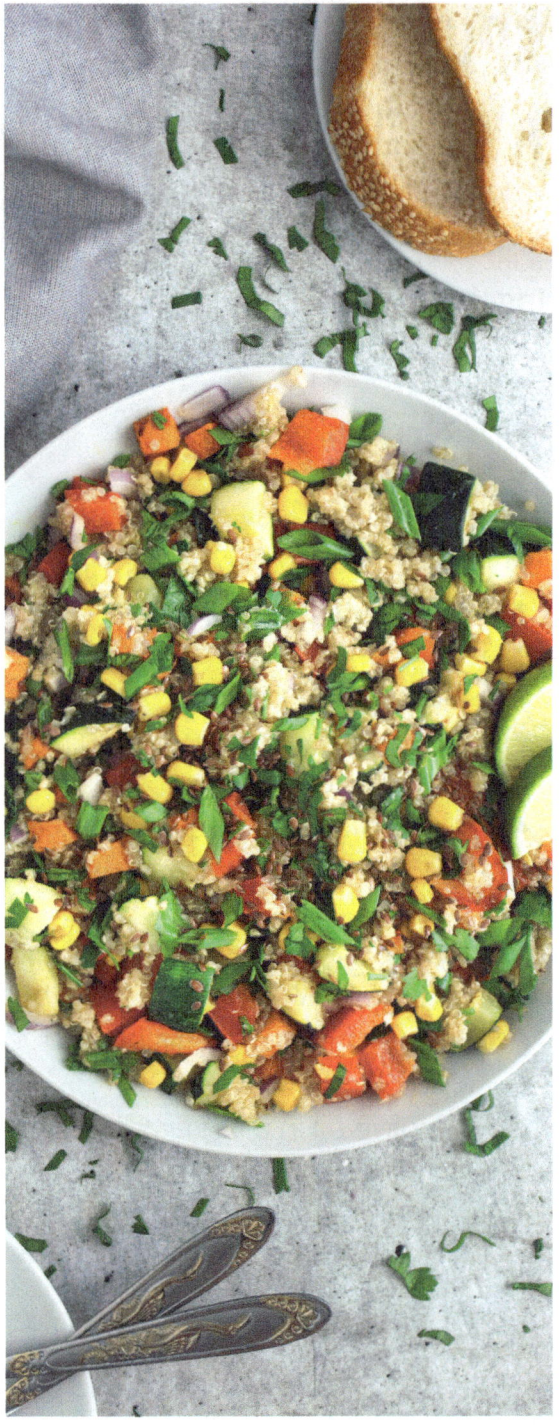

SAUTÉED SHRIMP WITH ZUCCHINI NOODLES AND PESTO

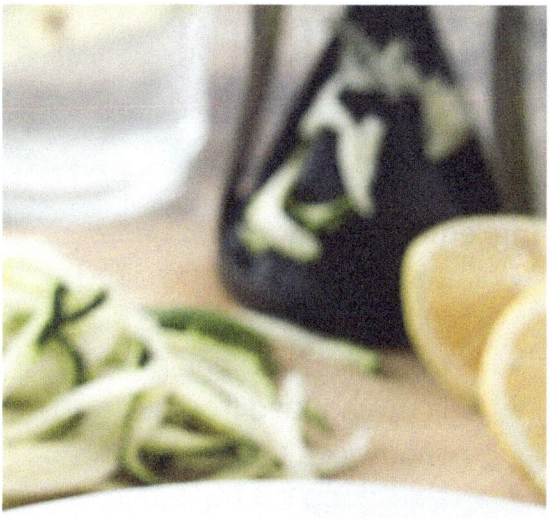

Ingredients:
- 1 tablespoon olive oil
- 1/2 pound uncooked shrimp, peeled and deveined
- salt and pepper to taste
- 2 cloves garlic, minced
- 2 zucchini, spiralized into noodles
- 1/4 cup pesto

Instructions:
1. Heat olive oil in a large skillet over medium heat. Add the shrimp, salt, pepper, and garlic. Cook until shrimp are opaque, about three minutes per side.
2. Add zucchini noodles and pesto to the skillet. Toss to combine. Cook for two minutes, or until zucchini noodles are slightly wilted.

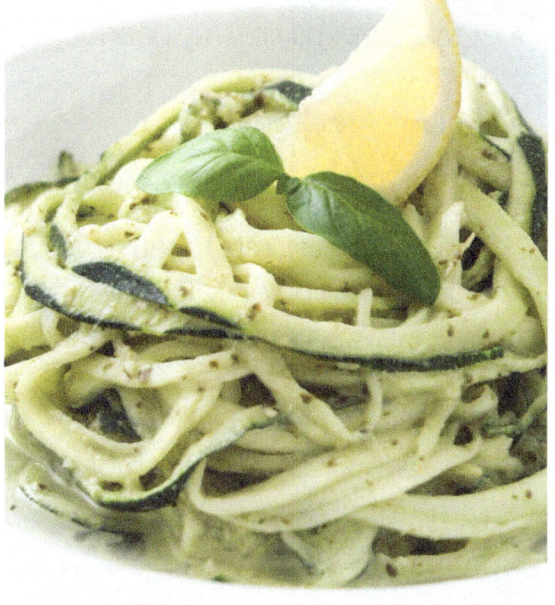

Serving size: 1/2 pound shrimp and 2 cups zucchini noodles
Calories: 400

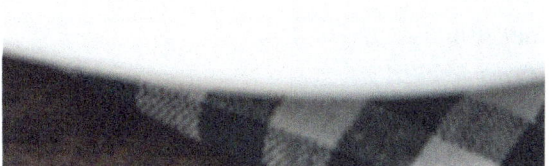

THAI CHICKEN WRAPS

Ingredients:
- 2 cups cooked and shredded chicken
- 1/4 cup diced red onion
- 1/4 cup chopped fresh cilantro
- 1/4 cup diced mango
- 1 tablespoon freshly squeezed lime juice
- salt and pepper to taste
- 2 tablespoons creamy peanut butter
- 4 gluten-free tortillas

Instructions:
1. In a large bowl, mix together cooked chicken, red onion, cilantro, mango, lime juice, salt, pepper, and peanut butter.
2. Lay out each tortilla. Divide the chicken mixture evenly among each tortilla. Roll them up and serve immediately.

Serving size: 1 wrap
Calories: 340

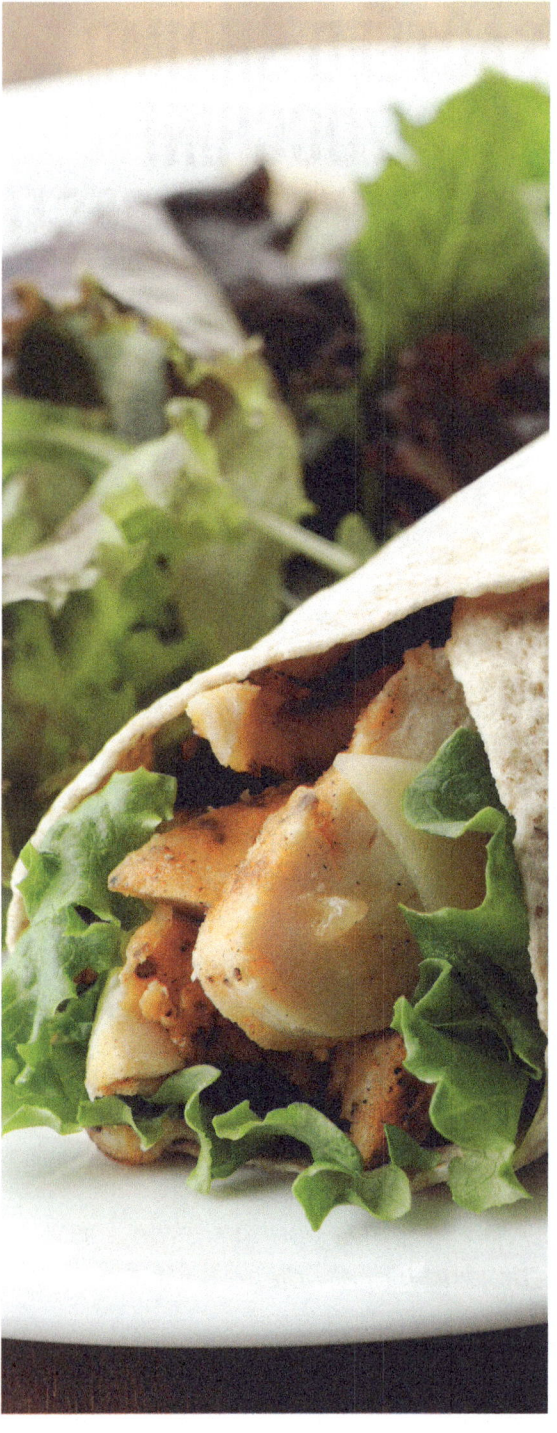

TURKEY AND APPLE SANDWICH ON GLUTEN-FREE BREAD

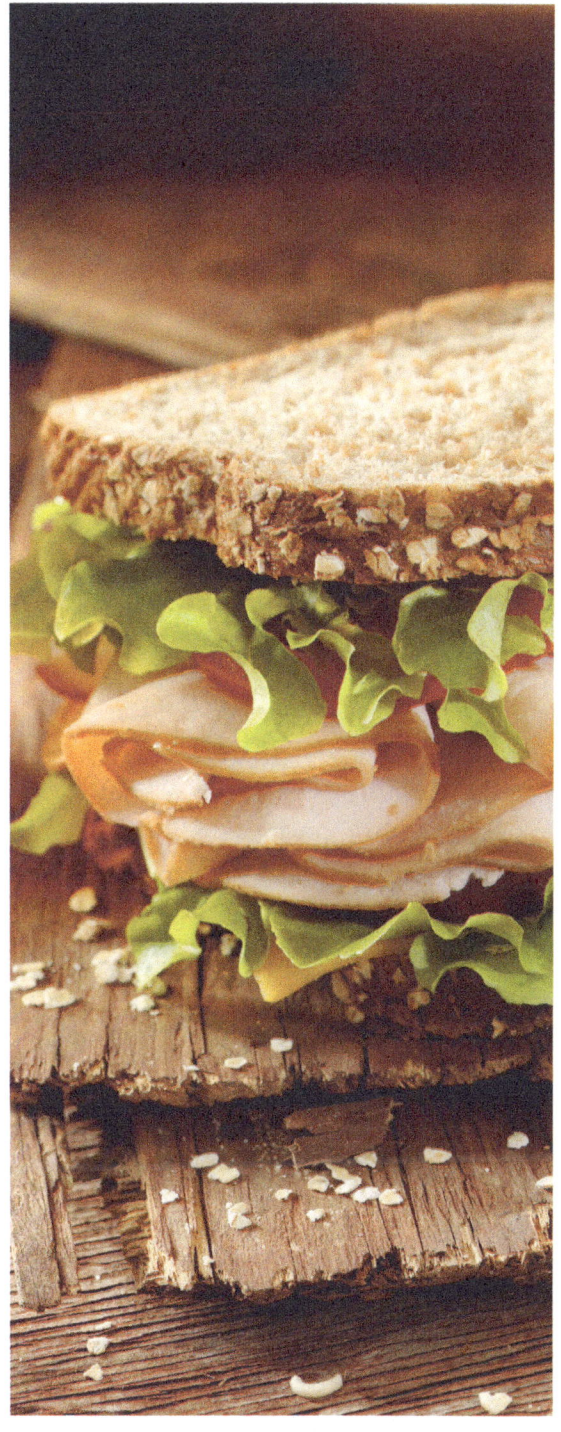

Ingredients:
- 2 slices gluten-free bread
- 2 tablespoons Dijon mustard
- 4 ounces thinly sliced turkey breast
- 1/2 green apple, thinly sliced
- 1/4 cup shredded Swiss cheese

Instructions:
1. Spread Dijon mustard on one slice of bread.
2. Top with turkey, apple slices, Swiss cheese, and the other slice of bread.
3. Serve immediately or wrap in wax paper and aluminum foil for a portable lunch.

Serving size: 1 sandwich
Calories: 440

SPAGHETTI SQUASH WITH TOMATO SAUCE

Ingredients:
- 1 spaghetti squash, halved lengthwise and seeded
- 1/2 cup water
- 1 jar (24 oz) marinara sauce

Instructions:
1. Preheat oven to 375 degrees F (190 degrees C).
2. Place the squash halves cut side down in a baking dish. Add the water. Cover and bake for about 30 minutes, until tender.
3. Scoop out the flesh of the squash with a fork, and place it in a bowl. Mix in the tomato sauce.

Serving size: 1/2 cup
Calories: 220

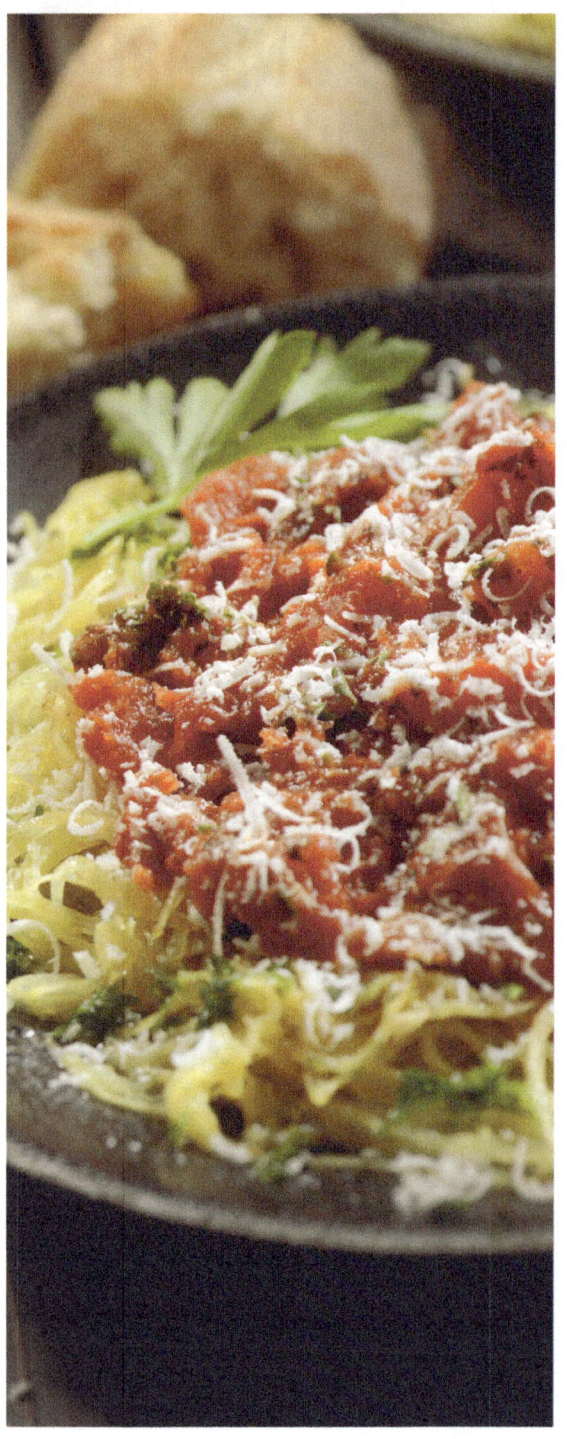

EGGPLANT PARMESAN

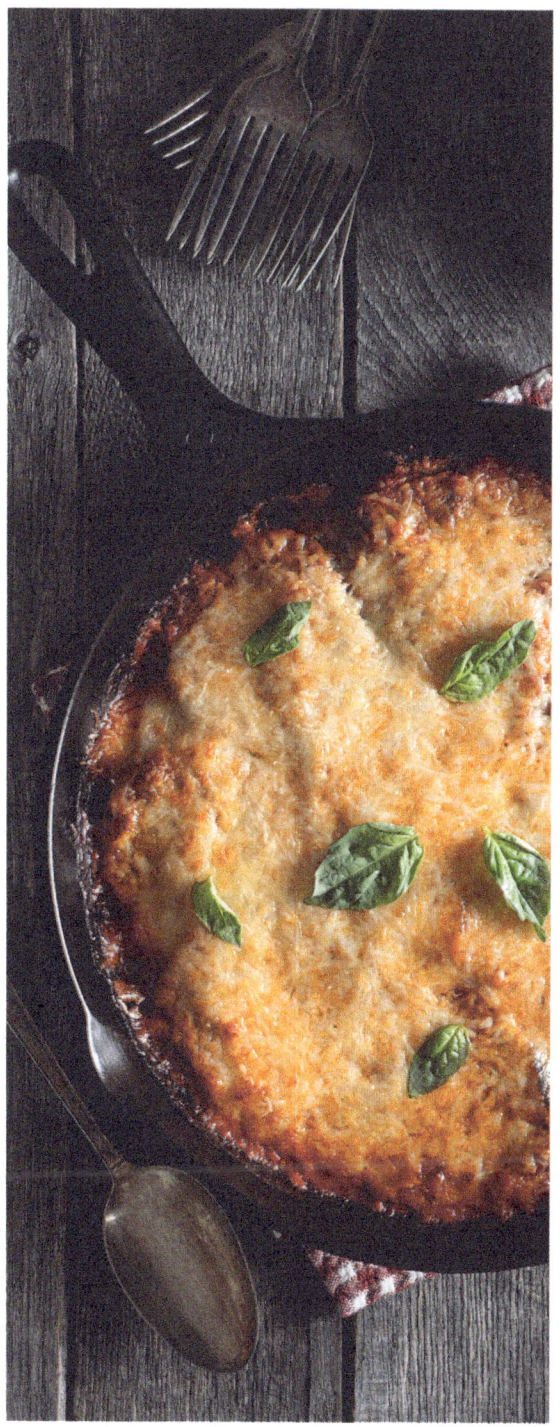

Ingredients:
- 1 large eggplant, sliced into 1/2-inch rounds
- 1/4 cup olive oil
- Salt and pepper to taste
- 2 cups marinara sauce
- 1 cup shredded mozzarella cheese

Instructions:
1. Preheat oven to 375 degrees F (190 degrees C).
2. Brush the eggplant slices with olive oil and season with salt and pepper. Place the eggplant on a baking sheet and bake for about 20 minutes, until tender.
3. In a 9x13 inch baking dish, spread 1 cup of marinara sauce on the bottom. Layer the eggplant slices over the sauce, and spread the remaining sauce on top. Sprinkle with mozzarella cheese.

Serving size: 1/2 eggplant round
Calories: 180

TURKEY WRAP

Ingredients:
- 2 ounces deli turkey breast, thinly sliced
- 1/4 avocado, mashed
- 1 tablespoon plain Greek yogurt
- 1 gluten-free tortilla wrap

Instructions:
1. Lay the tortilla wrap flat. In the center, spread the avocado, yogurt, and turkey slices. Roll up the wrap, cut in half, and serve.

Serving size: 1 wrap
Calories: 340

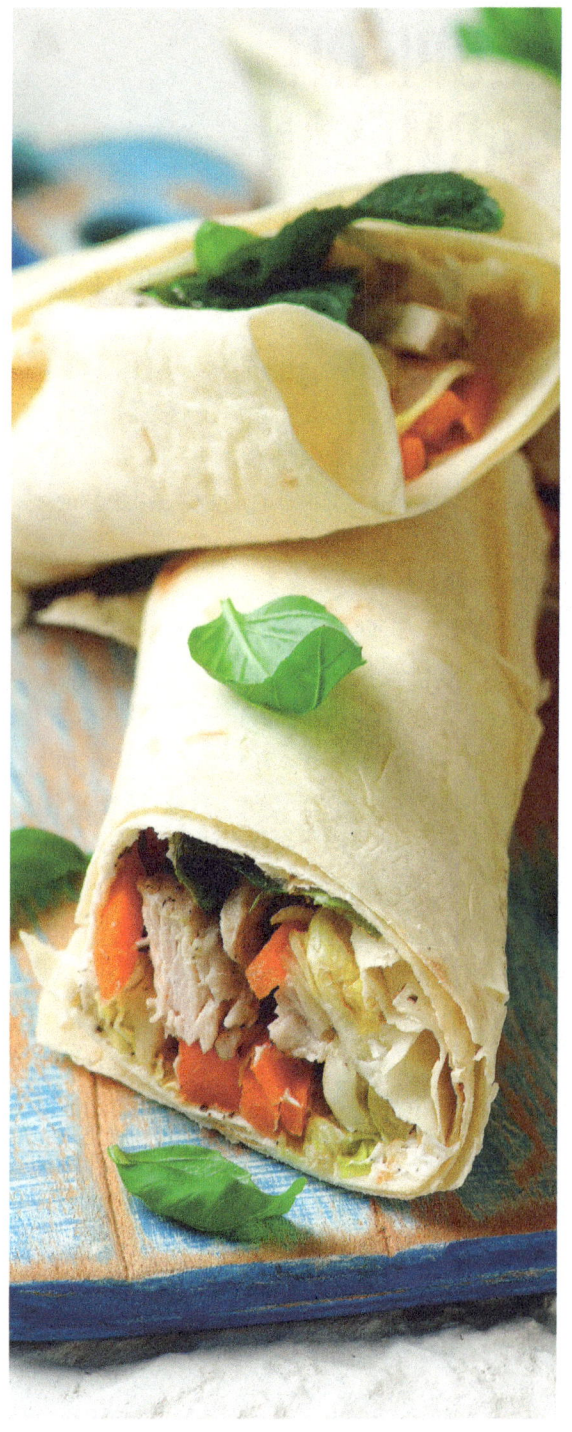

QUINOA PILAF

Ingredients:
- 1 tablespoon olive oil
- 1 onion, diced
- 1 cup uncooked quinoa, rinsed and drained
- 2 cups vegetable broth
- 1 can (15 oz) black beans, rinsed and drained
- 1/2 red bell pepper, diced
- 1/4 cup chopped fresh cilantro

Instructions:
1. In a large pot, heat the oil over medium heat. Add the onion and quinoa and cook for about 5 minutes, until the onion is soft.
2. Add the broth and bring to a boil. Reduce heat to low and simmer for about 15 minutes, until the quinoa is cooked.
3. Stir in the black beans, bell pepper, and cilantro.

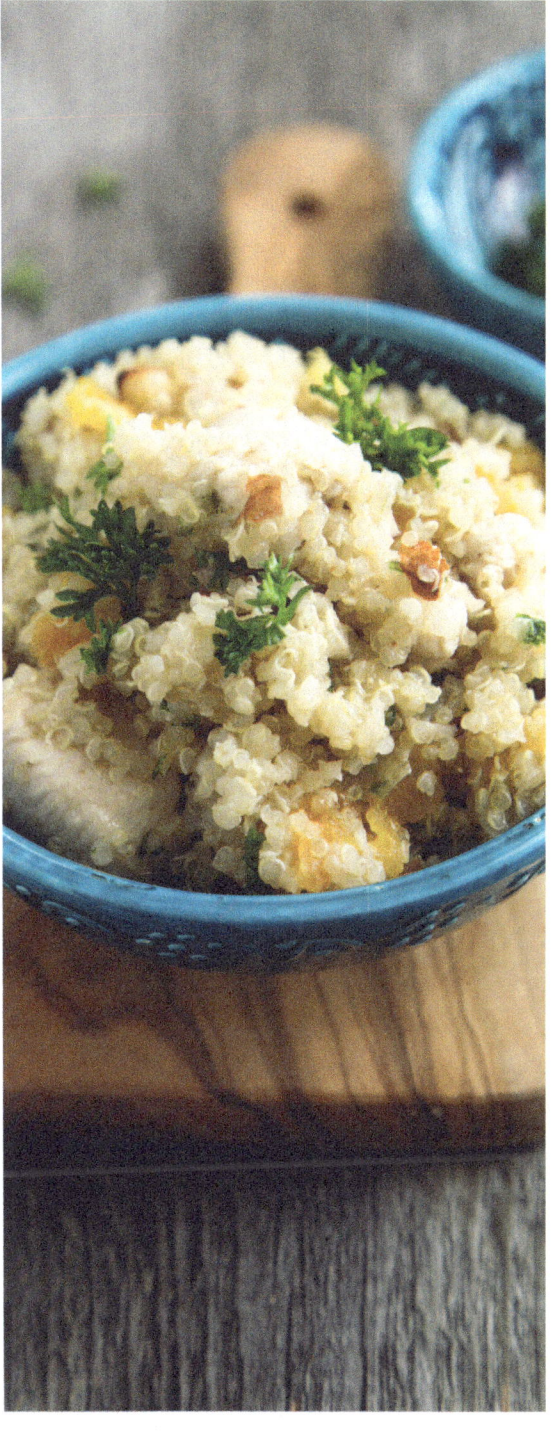

Serving size: 1 cup
Calories: 290

CHICKPEA SALAD

Ingredients:
- 1 can (15 oz) chickpeas, rinsed and drained
- 1/4 red onion, diced
- 1/4 cup diced celery
- 1/4 cup diced red grapes
- 1 tablespoon white wine vinegar
- 1 tablespoon olive oil
- Salt and pepper to taste

Instructions:
1. In a large bowl, mix together the chickpeas, onion, celery, grapes, vinegar, oil, salt, and pepper.

Serving size: 1 cup
Calories: 190

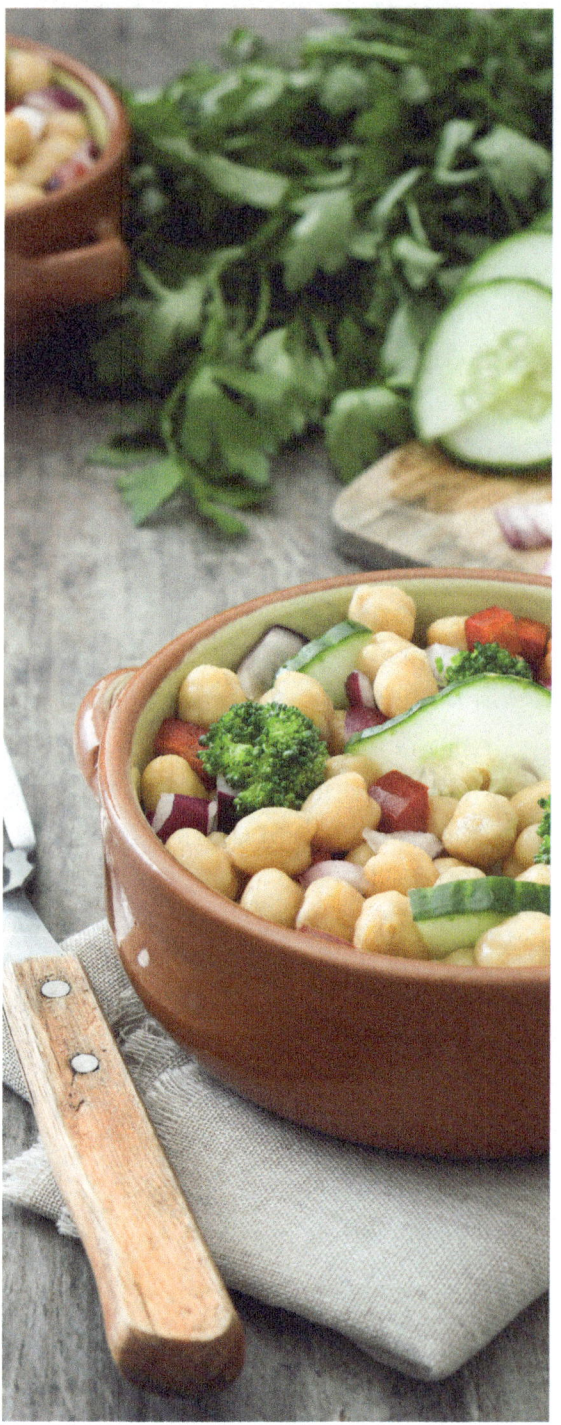

GARLIC MASHED POTATOES

Ingredients:
- 1 1/2 pounds potatoes, peeled and cubed
- 1/4 cup milk
- 3 tablespoons butter
- 1 clove garlic, minced
- Salt and pepper to taste

Instructions:
1. Place the potatoes in a pot and cover with water. Bring to a boil and cook for about 15 minutes, until tender. Drain.
2. In the same pot, heat the milk, butter, and garlic over low heat until the butter is melted. Add the cooked potatoes and mash until desired consistency is reached. Season with salt and pepper.

Serving size: 1 cup
Calories: 210

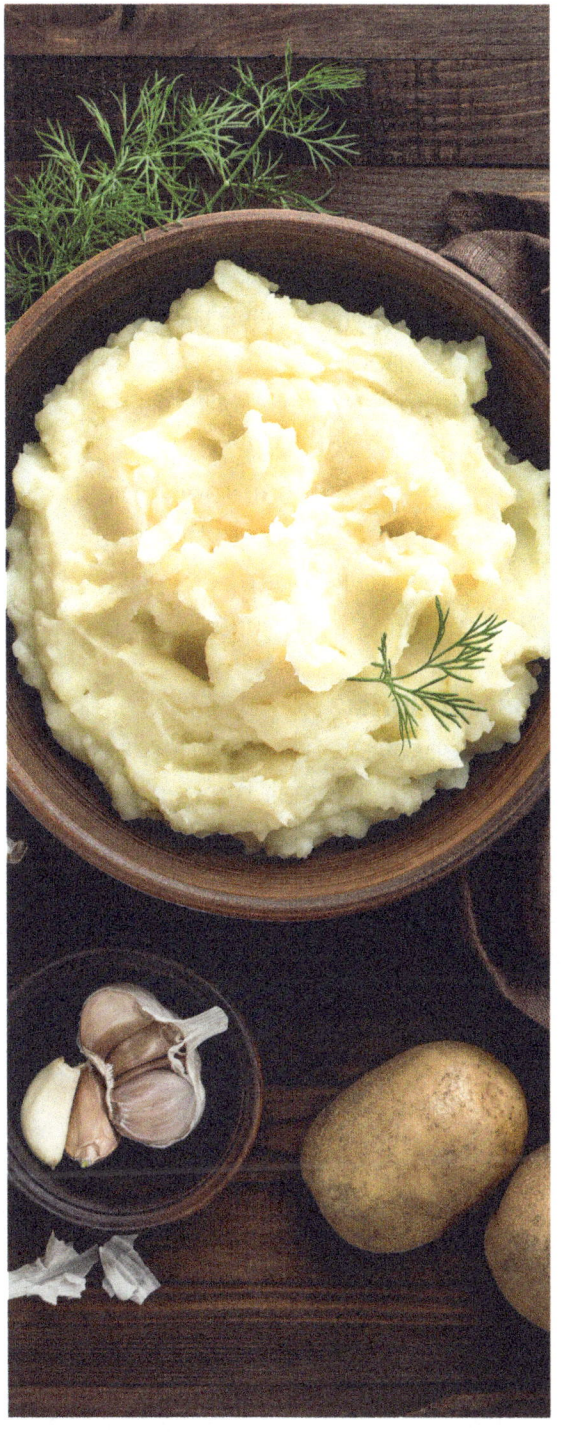

MEAT AND VEGETABLE ROLLUPS

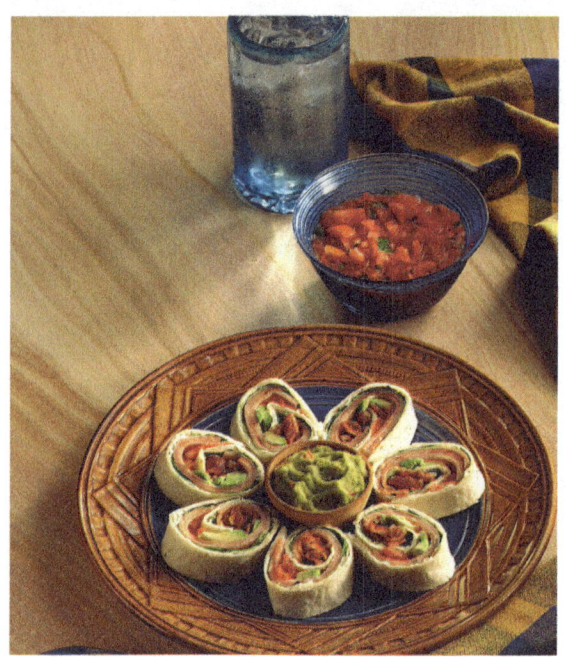

Ingredients:
- 1 pound thinly sliced flank steak
- 2 tablespoons olive oil
- 1 teaspoon garlic powder
- salt and pepper to taste
- 1 large zucchini
- 1 large yellow summer squash
- 4 ounces sliced mushrooms
- 2 roasted red peppers
- 8 gluten-free tortillas

Instructions:
1. Preheat oven to 350 degrees F (175 degrees C).
2. In a large resealable bag, combine the steak, olive oil, garlic powder, salt, and pepper. Seal bag and turn to coat. Set aside.
3. In a large skillet over medium-high heat, cook the zucchini, summer squash, mushrooms, and roasted red peppers until tender.
4. Lay out the tortillas. Divide the meat among them, then top with the vegetables. Roll up and serve.

Serving size: 1 rollup
Calories: 259

GARDEN VEGGIE SOUP

Ingredients:
- 1 tablespoon olive oil
- 1 onion, diced
- 3 cloves garlic, minced
- 4 cups vegetable broth
- 1 (14.5 ounce) can diced tomatoes, undrained
- 1 cup uncooked pearl couscous
- 1 zucchini, diced
- 1 yellow summer squash, diced
- 1 green bell pepper, diced
- 2 carrots, diced
- salt and pepper to taste

Instructions:
1. In a large pot over medium heat, heat the olive oil. Add the onion and garlic, and cook until softened.
2. Stir in the vegetable broth, tomatoes, couscous, zucchini, summer squash, bell pepper, carrots, salt, and pepper. Bring to a boil. Reduce heat to low and simmer for 20 minutes, or until the vegetables are tender and the couscous is cooked.

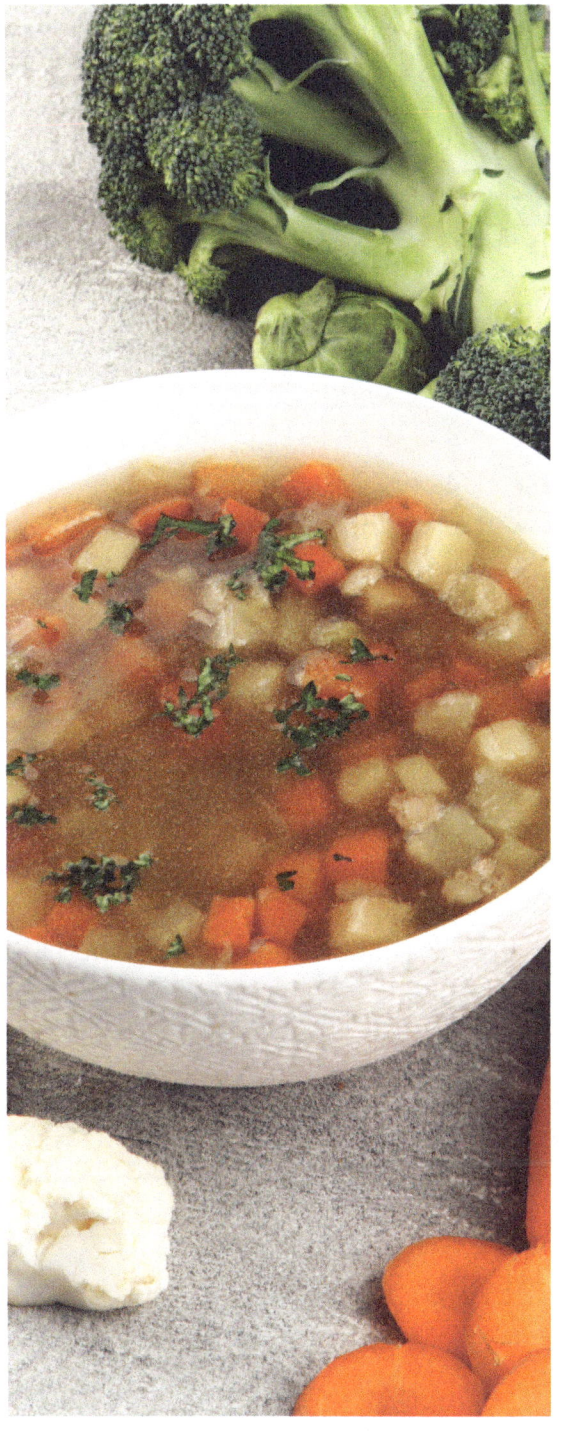

Serving size: 1 bowl
Calories:292

QUINOA SALAD WITH CRANBERRIES AND FETA

Ingredients:
- 1 cup uncooked quinoa
- 2 cups water
- 1/4 cup white balsamic vinegar
- 1/4 cup olive oil
- 1 tablespoon honey
- salt and pepper to taste
- 1/2 cup dried cranberries
- 1/2 cup crumbled feta cheese
- 1/4 cup chopped pecans, toasted

Instructions:
1. In a large saucepan, bring the quinoa and water to a boil. Reduce heat to low and simmer for about 15 minutes, or until the quinoa is cooked.
2. In a small bowl, whisk together the vinegar, olive oil, honey, salt, and pepper.
3. In a large bowl, combine the cooked quinoa, cranberries, feta cheese, pecans, and dressing. Toss to combine.

Serving size: 1/2 cup
Calories: 220

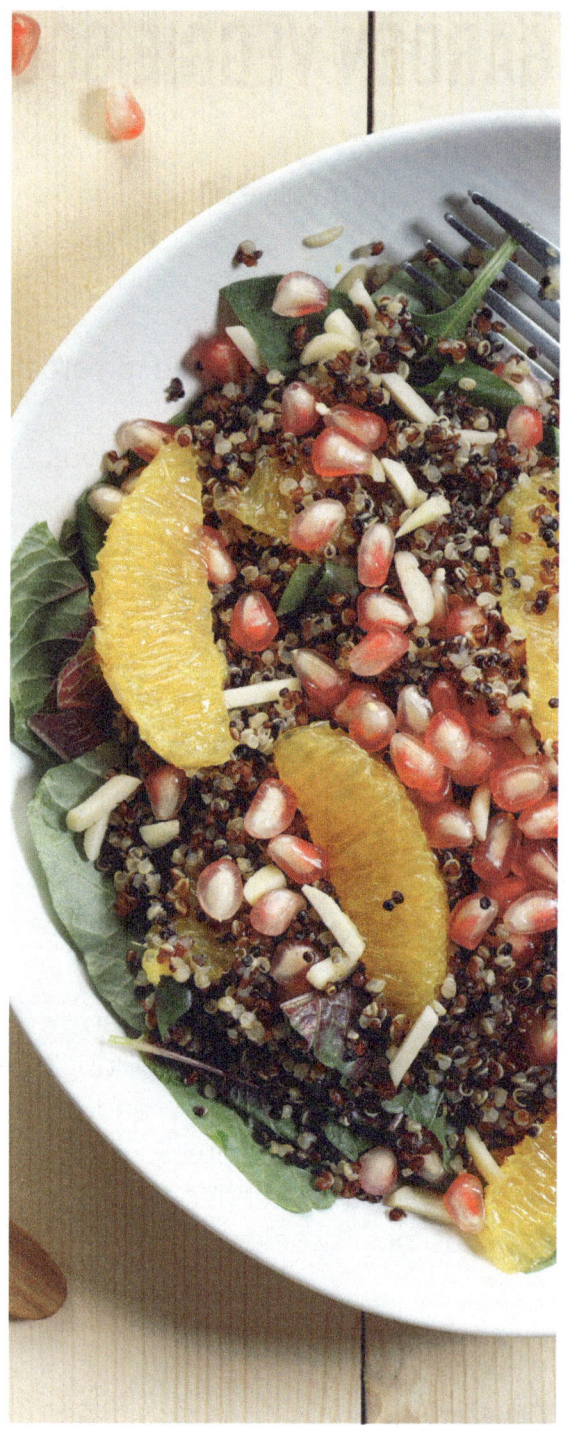

POTATO SOUP WITH BACON, CHEESE, AND SCALLIONS

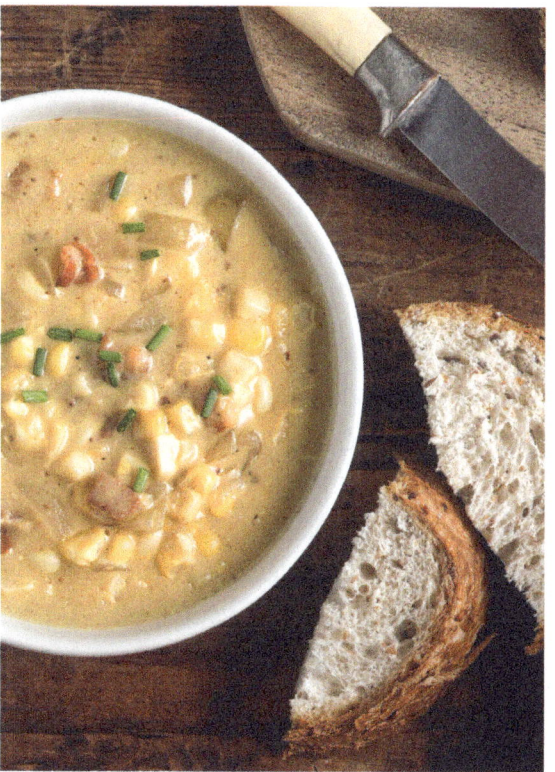

Ingredients:
- 6 slices bacon, diced
- 1 onion, diced
- 3 cloves garlic, minced
- 6 potatoes, peeled and cubed
- 4 cups chicken broth
- salt and pepper to taste
- 1 cup shredded Cheddar cheese
- 2 tablespoons chopped fresh parsley
- 4 scallions, thinly sliced

Instructions:
1. In a large pot over medium heat, cook the bacon until crisp. Remove with a slotted spoon and drain on paper towels.
2. In the same pot, add the onion and garlic. Cook until softened.
3. Stir in the potatoes and chicken broth. Season with salt and pepper. Bring to a boil. Reduce heat to low and simmer for 20 minutes, or until the potatoes are tender.
4. Stir in the bacon, cheese, parsley, and scallions. Cook for 5 minutes, or until the cheese is melted.

Serving size: 1 cup
Calories: 290

PINK SALMON SALAD WITH VEGETABLES

Ingredients:
- 2 (6 ounce) cans pink salmon, drained and flaked
- 1/4 cup mayonnaise
- 1/4 cup sour cream
- 1 tablespoon lemon juice
- salt and pepper to taste
- 2 stalks celery, diced
- 1/4 cup chopped red onion
- 1/4 cup chopped green bell pepper
- lettuce leaves
- 1 tomato, sliced

Instructions:
1. In a medium bowl, combine the salmon, mayonnaise, sour cream, lemon juice, salt, and pepper. Stir in the celery, red onion, and green bell pepper.
2. Place the lettuce leaves on a plate. Top with the salmon salad and tomato slices.

Serving size: 1 salad
Calories: 320

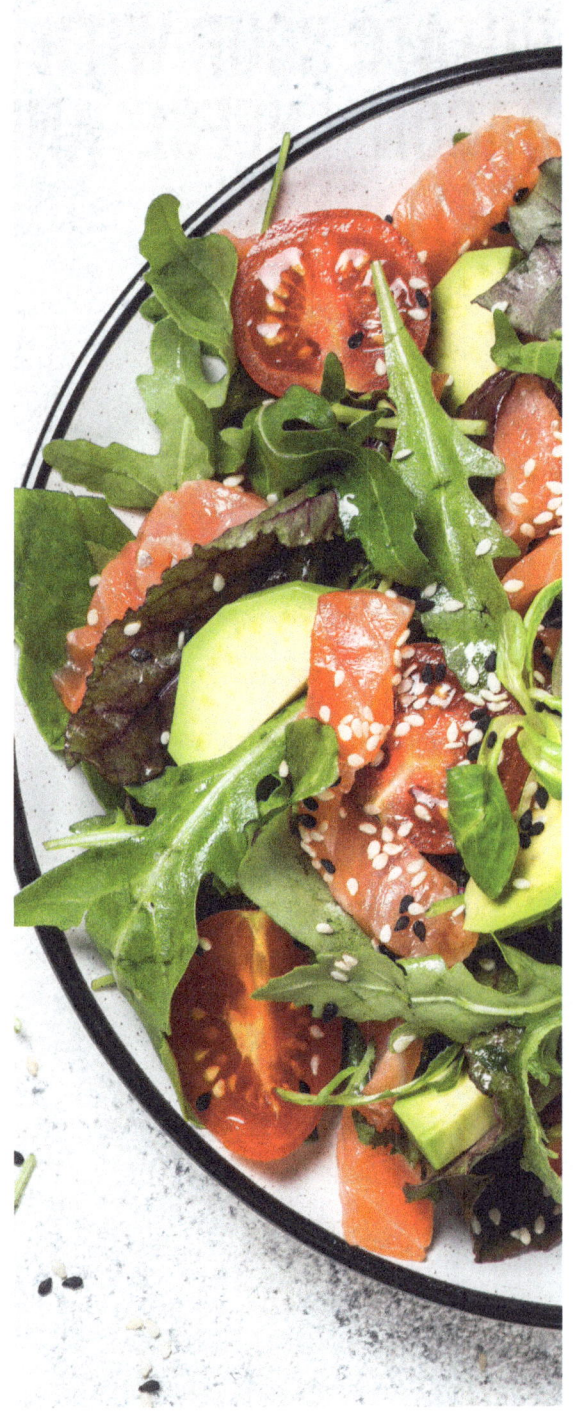

SPICY SAUSAGE AND KALE SOUP

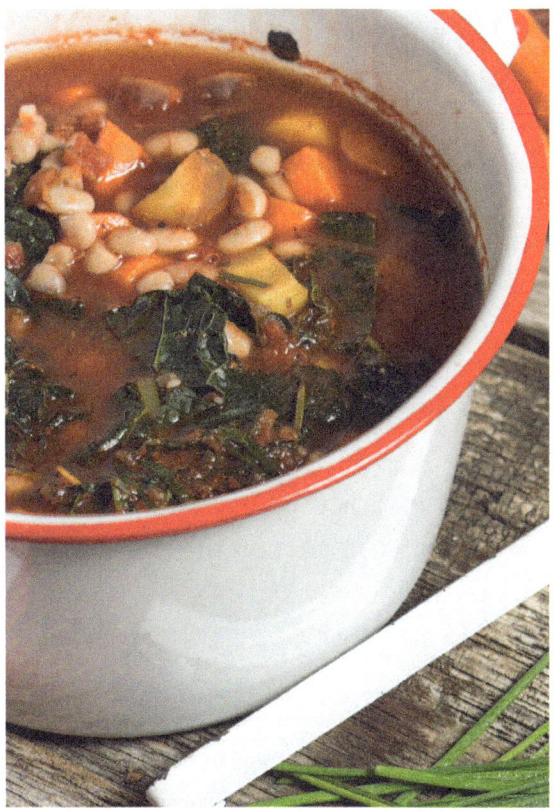

Ingredients:
- 1 tablespoon olive oil
- 1 pound hot Italian sausage
- 1 onion, diced
- 3 cloves garlic, minced
- 4 cups chicken broth
- 1 (14.5 ounce) can diced tomatoes, undrained
- 1 teaspoon dried oregano
- 1/4 teaspoon crushed red pepper flakes
- salt and pepper to taste
- 1 bunch kale, stemmed and chopped

Instructions:
1. In a large pot over medium heat, heat the olive oil. Add the sausage, onion, and garlic. Cook until the sausage is browned.
2. Stir in the chicken broth, tomatoes, oregano, red pepper flakes, salt, and pepper. Bring to a boil. Reduce heat to low and simmer for 30 minutes, or until the kale is tender.

Serving size: 1 cup
Calories: 260

TOMATO BASIL CHICKEN

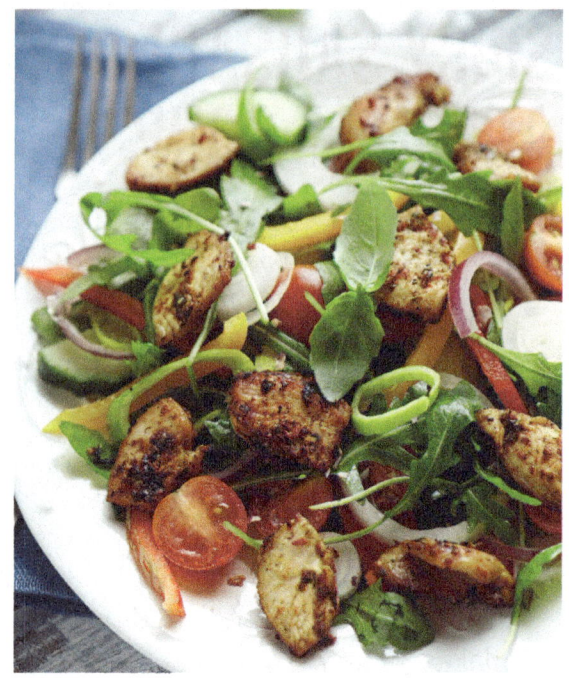

Ingredients:
- 4 chicken breasts, skinless and boneless
- salt and pepper to taste
- 1 tablespoon olive oil
- 3 cloves garlic, minced
- 1 onion, diced
- 1 (14.5 ounce) can diced tomatoes, undrained
- 1/4 cup chopped fresh basil leaves

Instructions:
1. Season the chicken breasts with salt and pepper.
2. In a large skillet over medium heat, heat the olive oil. Add the chicken and cook for about 5 minutes per side, or until golden brown.
3. Remove the chicken from the skillet and set aside.
4. To the same skillet, add the garlic, onion, tomatoes, and basil. Cook for 5 minutes, or until the onion is softened.
5. Return the chicken to the skillet. Cover and simmer for 10 minutes, or until the chicken is cooked through.

Serving size: 1 chicken breast
Calories: 280

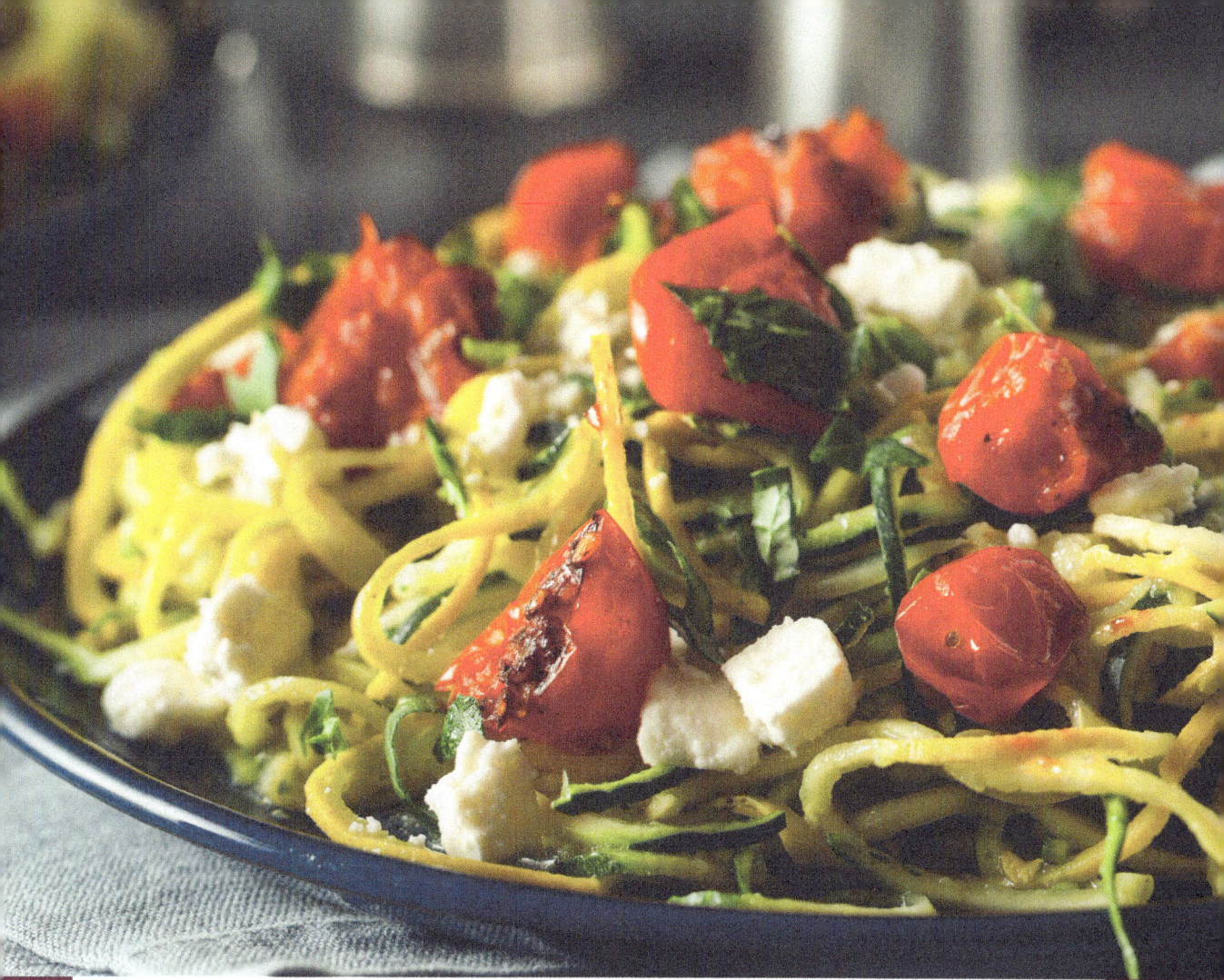

CHAPTER FIVE: DINNERS

CHICKEN AND BROCCOLI STIR FRY

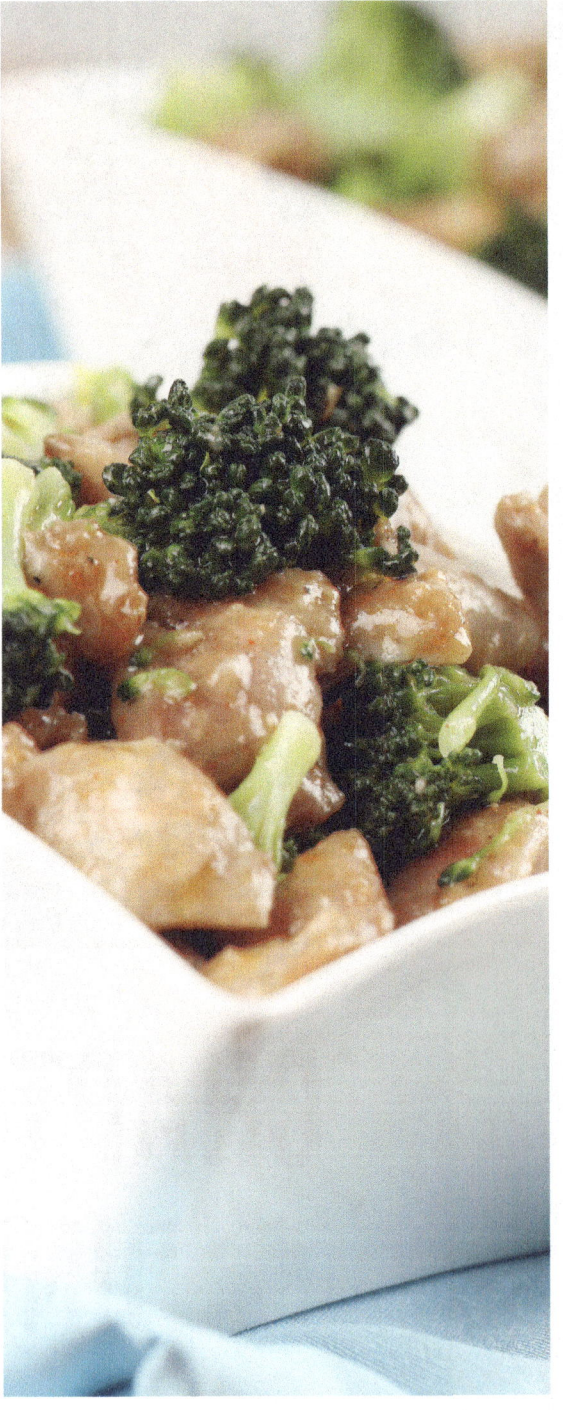

Ingredients:
- 1 lb. boneless, skinless chicken breast
- 2 cups broccoli florets
- 1/4 cup soy sauce
- 1 tbsp. Honey
- 1 tbsp. vegetable oil
- 1 clove garlic, minced
- salt and pepper to taste

Instructions:
1. Add all ingredients to a large bowl and mix together until well combined.
2. Pour mixture into a large skillet over medium-high heat.
3. Cook for 5-7 minutes per side or until chicken is cooked through and broccoli is tender.
4. Serve over rice or quinoa if desired!

Serving size: 1/2 cup
Calories: 495

GRILLED CHICKEN WITH ROASTED VEGETABLES

Ingredients:
- 1 lb. boneless, skinless chicken breast
- 1/2 lb. mixed vegetables (broccoli, carrots, peppers, etc.)
- 1 tbsp. olive oil
- salt and pepper to taste

Instructions:
1. Preheat grill to medium-high heat.
2. Season chicken and vegetables with olive oil, salt, and pepper.
3. Grill chicken for 5-7 minutes per side or until cooked through.
4. Add vegetables to grill basket or foil packet.
5. Grill for 10-12 minutes or until tender.
6. Serve chicken and vegetables together!

Serving size: 1/2 chicken breast and 1 cup vegetables
Calories: 400

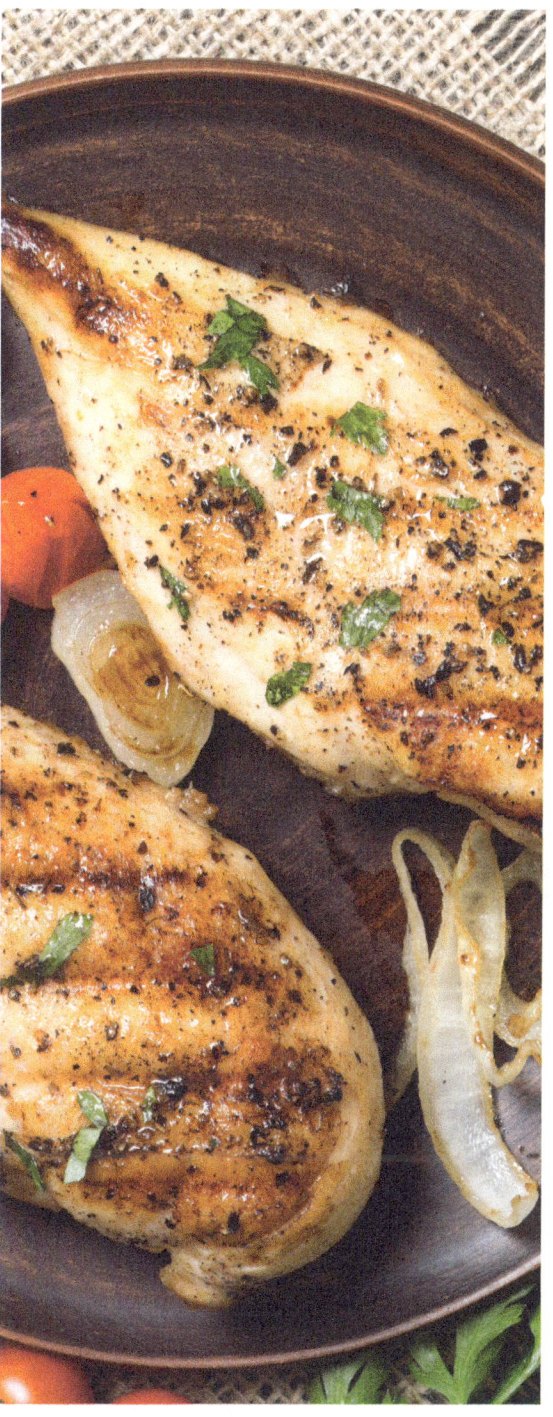

CROCKPOT HONEY GARLIC CHICKEN

Ingredients:
- 1 lb. boneless, skinless chicken breast
- 1/4 cup soy sauce
- 1/4 cup honey
- 3 cloves garlic, minced
- salt and pepper to taste

Instructions:
1. Add all ingredients to a crockpot and mix together until well combined.
2. Cook on low for 6-8 hours or on high for 3-4 hours.
3. Serve over rice or quinoa if desired!

Serving size: 1/2 chicken breast
Calories: 330

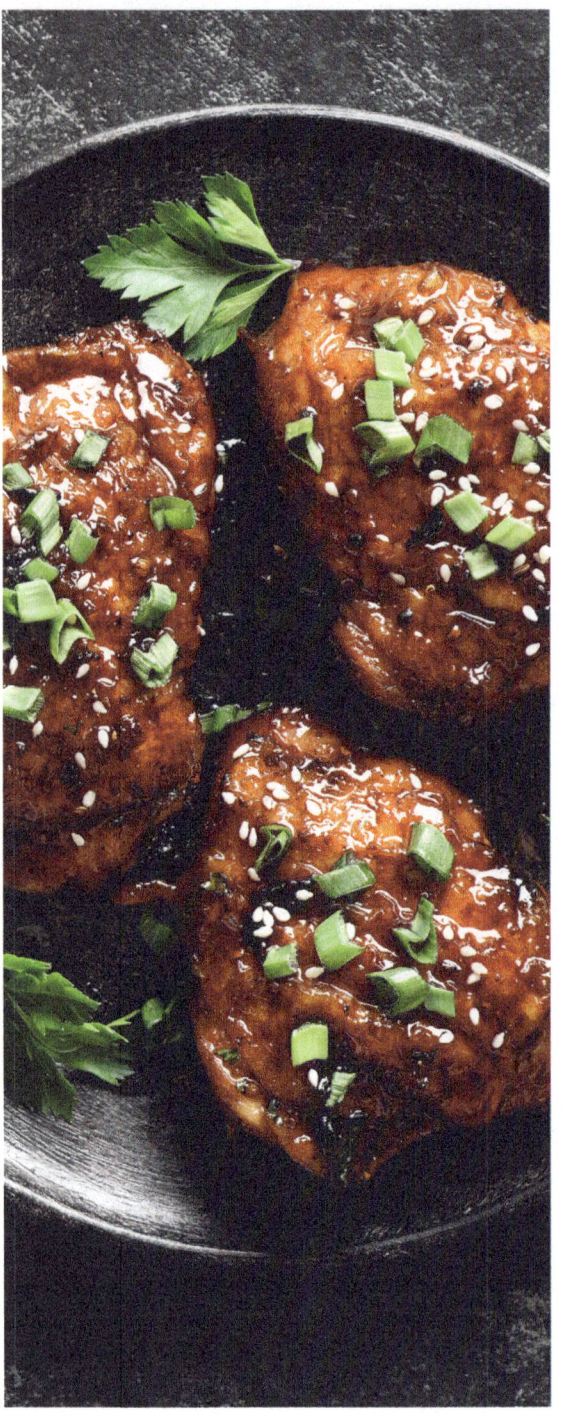

ONE POT BBQ CHICKEN AND QUINOA

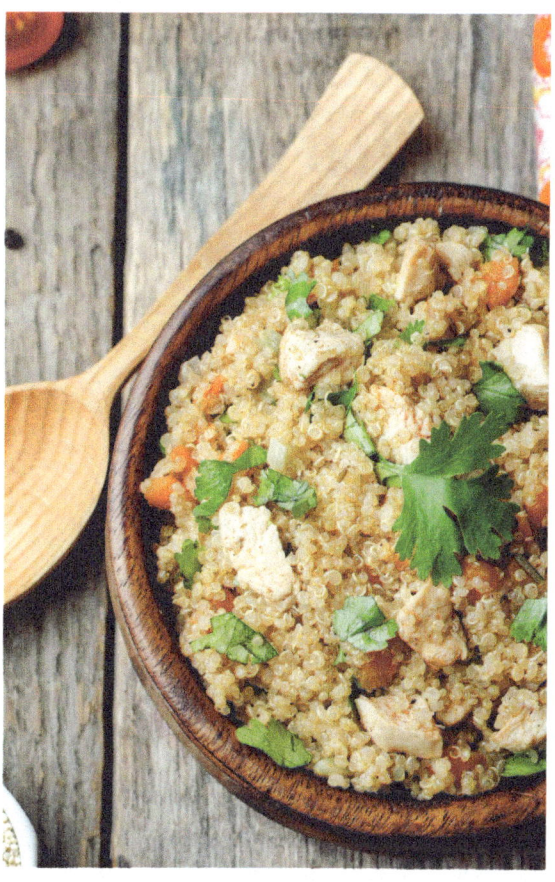

Ingredients:
- 1 lb. boneless, skinless chicken breast, diced into small pieces
- 1 cup quinoa, rinsed
- 1 (15 oz) can black beans, drained and rinsed
- 1 tbsp. chili powder
- 1 tsp. smoked paprika
- 1 tsp. cumin
- 1/2 tsp. garlic powder
- 1 cup salsa
- 2 cups chicken broth
- salt and pepper to taste

Instructions:
1. Add all ingredients to a large pot or Dutch oven and mix together until well combined.
2. Bring mixture to a boil then reduce heat to low and simmer for 15-20 minutes or until quinoa is fully cooked.
3. Serve as is or top with shredded cheese, sour cream, or green onions if desired!

Serving size: 1 cup
Calories: 490

SALMON WITH ROASTED BRUSSELS SPROUTS

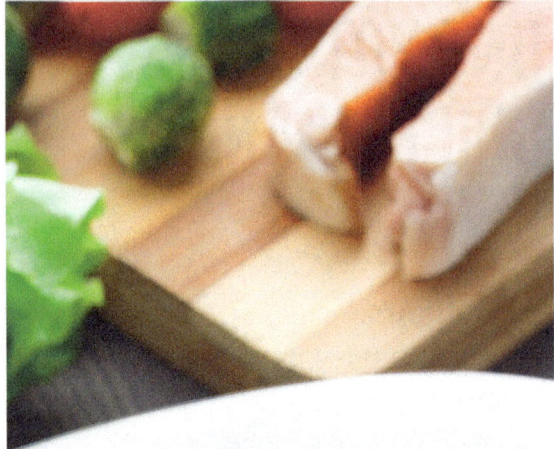

Ingredients:
- 1 lb. salmon
- 1 lb. Brussels sprouts
- 1 tbsp. olive oil
- salt and pepper to taste

Instructions:
1. Preheat oven to 400 degrees F.
2. Cut Brussels sprouts in half and toss with olive oil, salt, and pepper. Spread on one side of a baking sheet.
3. Place salmon filets on the other side of the baking sheet and season with salt and pepper.
4. Bake for 12-15 minutes or until salmon is cooked through and Brussels sprouts are slightly browned and tender.
5. Serve immediately!

Serving size: 1/2 salmon filet and 1 cup Brussels sprouts
Calories: 400

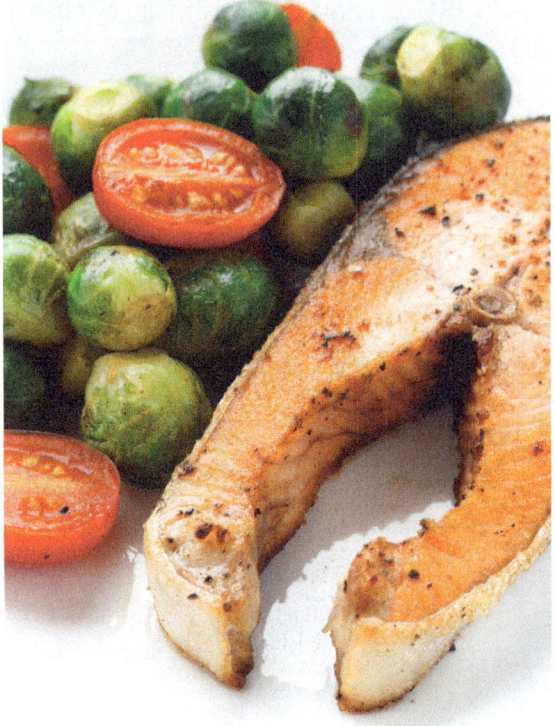

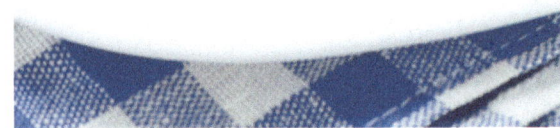

BEEF STIR FRY WITH BROCCOLI AND BROWN RICE

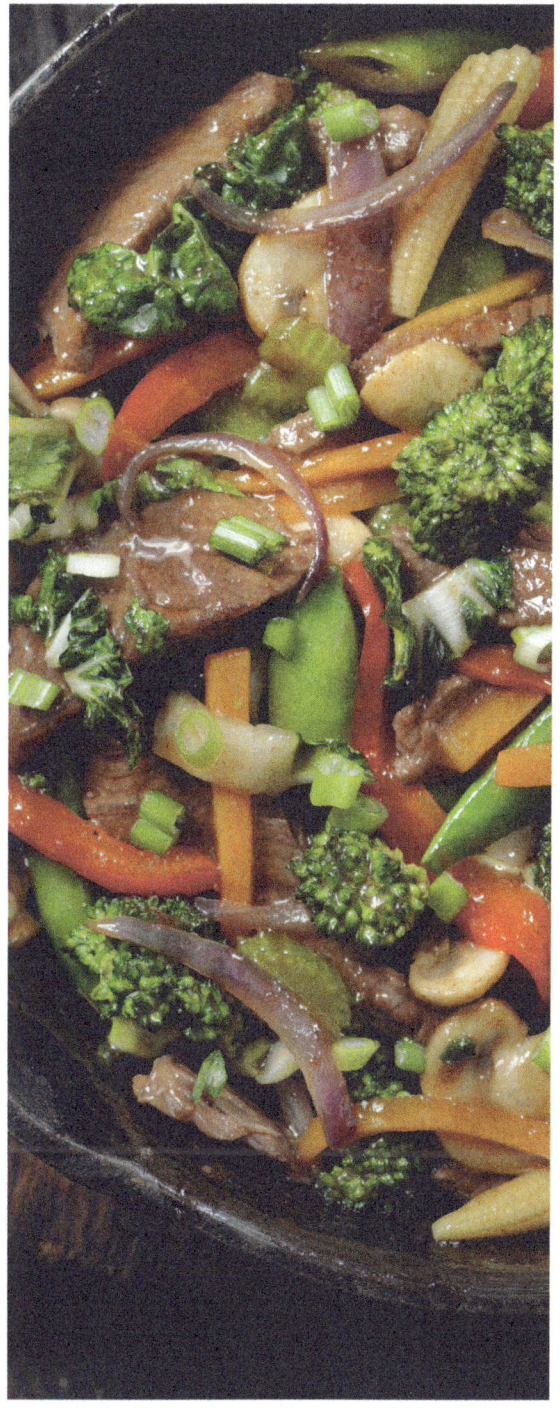

Ingredients:
- 1 lb. lean beef, thinly sliced
- 2 cups broccoli florets
- 1/4 cup soy sauce
- 1 tbsp. vegetable oil
- 3 cloves garlic, minced
- salt and pepper to taste

Instructions:
1. Add all ingredients to a large bowl and mix together until well combined.
2. Pour mixture into a large skillet over medium-high heat.
3. Cook for 5-7 minutes per side or until beef is cooked through and broccoli is tender.
4. Serve over brown rice if desired!

Serving size: 1/2 cup
Calories: 500

TURKEY BURGER WITH SWEET POTATO FRIES

Ingredients:
- 1 lb. ground turkey
- 1/4 cup bread crumbs
- 1 egg, beaten
- 1 tbsp. ketchup
- 1 tsp. mustard
- salt and pepper to taste

For the sweet potato fries:
- 2 large sweet potatoes, cut into fry-sized pieces
- 2 tbsp. olive oil
- salt and pepper to taste

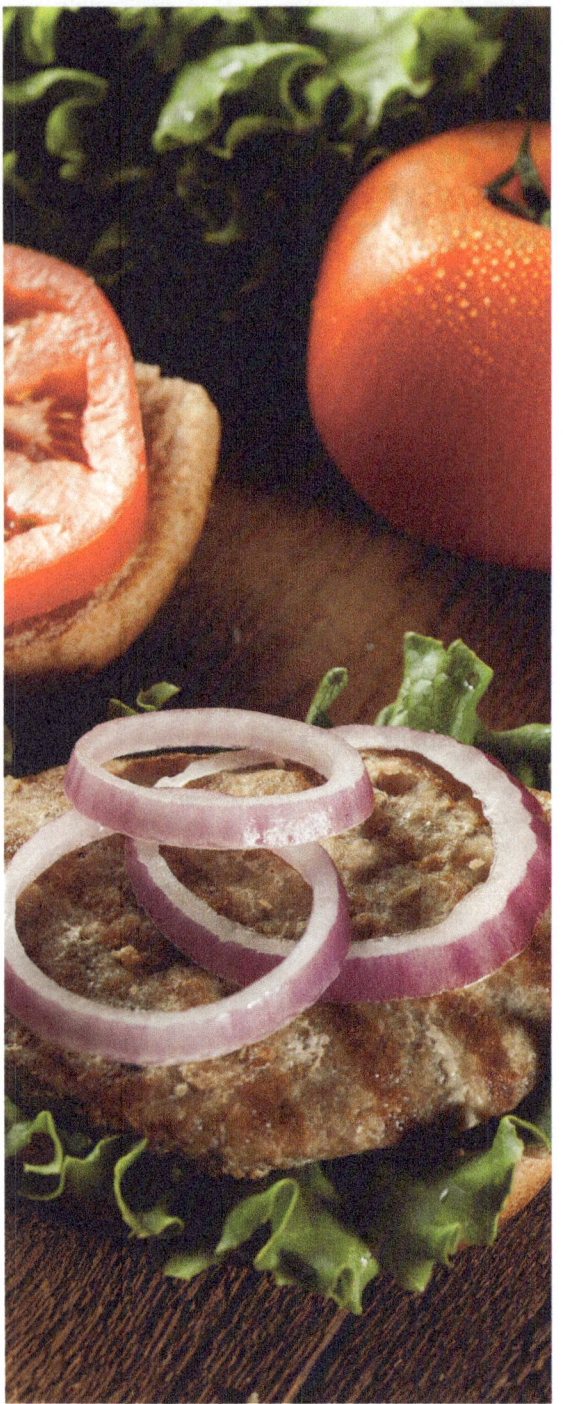

Instructions:
1. Preheat oven to 400 degrees F.
2. In a large bowl, mix together ground turkey, bread crumbs, egg, ketchup, mustard, salt, and pepper until well combined.
3. Form mixture into 4-6 patties and place on a baking sheet lined with foil or parchment paper. Bake for 15-20 minutes or until cooked through.
4. While burgers are cooking, toss sweet potato fries with olive oil, salt, and pepper. Spread on another baking sheet lined with foil or parchment paper.
5. Bake for 20-25 minutes or until tender and slightly browned.
6. Serve turkey burgers with sweet potato fries!

Serving size: 1 turkey burger and 1/2 cup sweet potato fries
Calories: 520

QUINOA SALAD WITH GRILLED CHICKEN

Ingredients:
- 1 cup quinoa, cooked according to package instructions
- 2 cups chopped kale
- 1/4 cup dried cranberries
- 1/4 cup slivered almonds
- 2 tbsp. olive oil
- 3 cloves garlic, minced
- salt and pepper to taste

For the grilled chicken:
- 1 lb. boneless, skinless chicken breast
- 1 tsp. chili powder
- 1 tsp. smoked paprika
- 1/2 tsp. garlic powder
- salt and pepper to taste

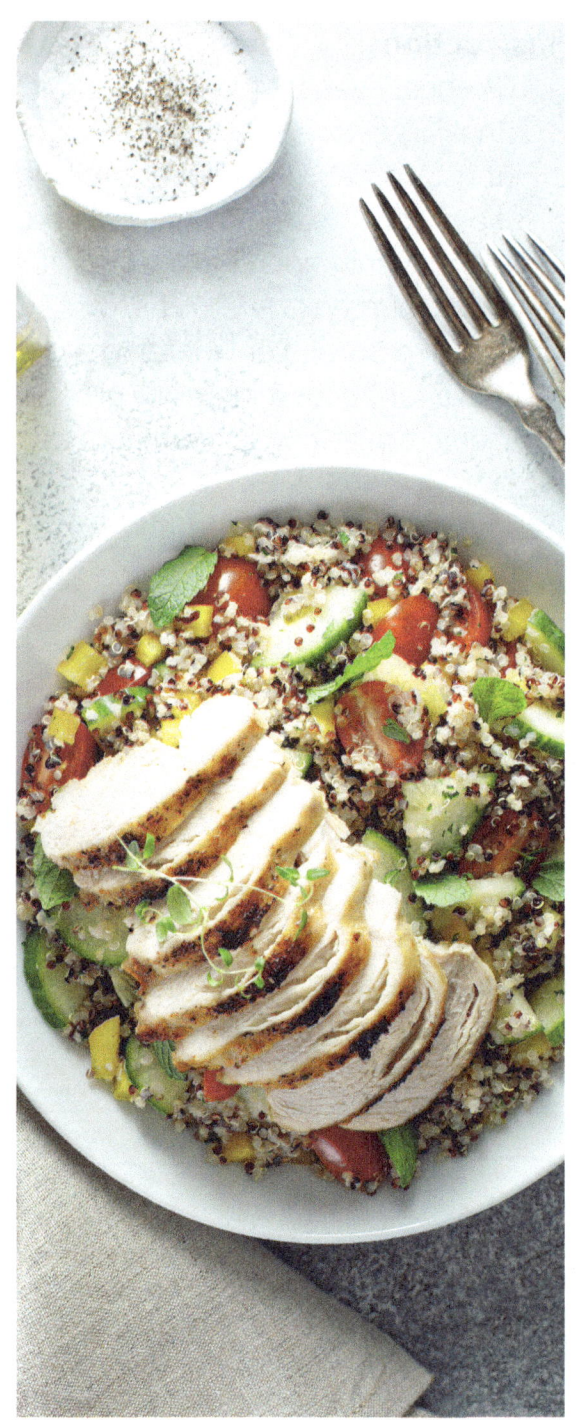

Matthew Thrush

Instructions:
1. Preheat grill to medium-high heat.
2. In a large bowl, mix together quinoa, kale, cranberries, slivered almonds, olive oil, garlic, salt, and pepper until well combined.
3. Season chicken breasts with chili powder, smoked paprika, garlic powder, salt and pepper then place on the grill. Grill for 5-7 minutes per side or until cooked through.
4. Remove from grill and chop into bite-sized pieces.
5. Add grilled chicken to quinoa salad and mix together until well combined. Serve immediately!

Serving size: 1 cup
Calories: 530

LENTIL SOUP

Ingredients:
- 1 lb. lentils, rinsed and drained
- 8 cups chicken or vegetable broth
- 2 carrots, diced
- 2 stalks celery, diced
- 1 onion, diced
- 3 cloves garlic, minced
- 1 tbsp. olive oil
- salt and pepper to taste

Instructions:
1. In a large pot or Dutch oven, heat olive oil over medium heat.
2. Add onions, carrots, celery, and garlic and cook until vegetables are soft and translucent.
3. Add lentils and chicken broth and bring to a boil.
4. Reduce heat to low and simmer for 30-45 minutes or until lentils are soft.
5. Season with salt and pepper to taste. Serve immediately!

Serving size: 1 cup
Calories: 540

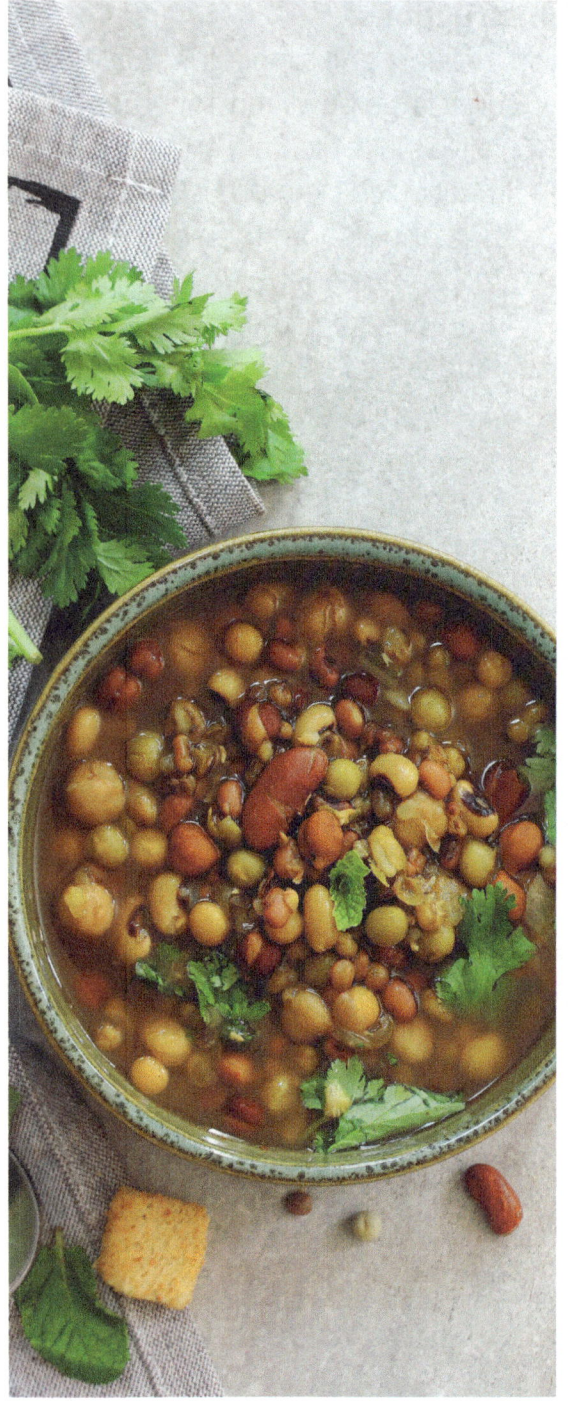

SPAGHETTI SQUASH WITH TURKEY MEAT SAUCE

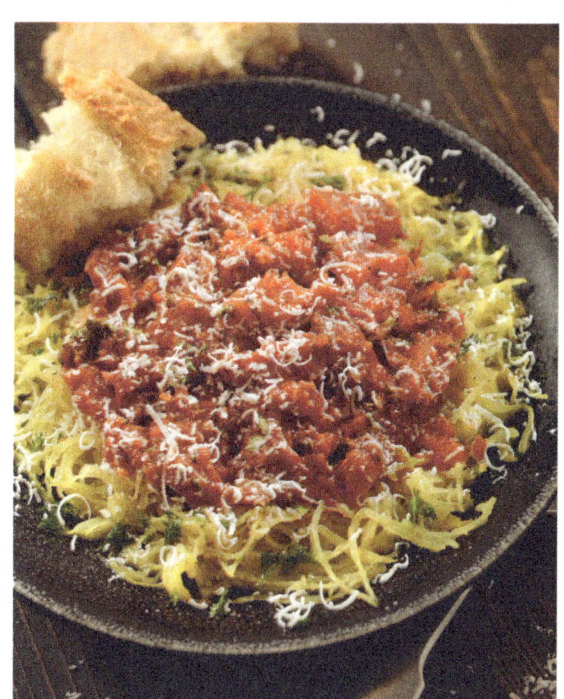

Ingredients:
- 1 large spaghetti squash, halved lengthwise and seeded
- 1 lb. lean ground turkey
- 1 can (28 oz.) crushed tomatoes
- 2 cloves garlic, minced
- 1 onion, diced
- 1 tbsp. olive oil
- salt and pepper to taste

Instructions:
1. Preheat oven to 375 degrees F.
2. In a large skillet, heat olive oil over medium-high heat.
3. Add onions and garlic and cook until soft and translucent.
4. Add ground turkey and cook until browned.
5. Stir in crushed tomatoes and bring to a simmer. Simmer for 10 minutes or until slightly thickened.
6. Season with salt and pepper to taste.
7. Place spaghetti squash halves cut side up on a baking sheet lined with foil or parchment paper. Spoon meat sauce evenly over each half.
8. Bake for 30-40 minutes or until squash is tender when pierced with a fork. Serve immediately!

Serving size: 1/2 spaghetti squash with 1/2 cup meat sauce
Calories: 550

ROASTED CHICKEN WITH ROASTED VEGETABLES

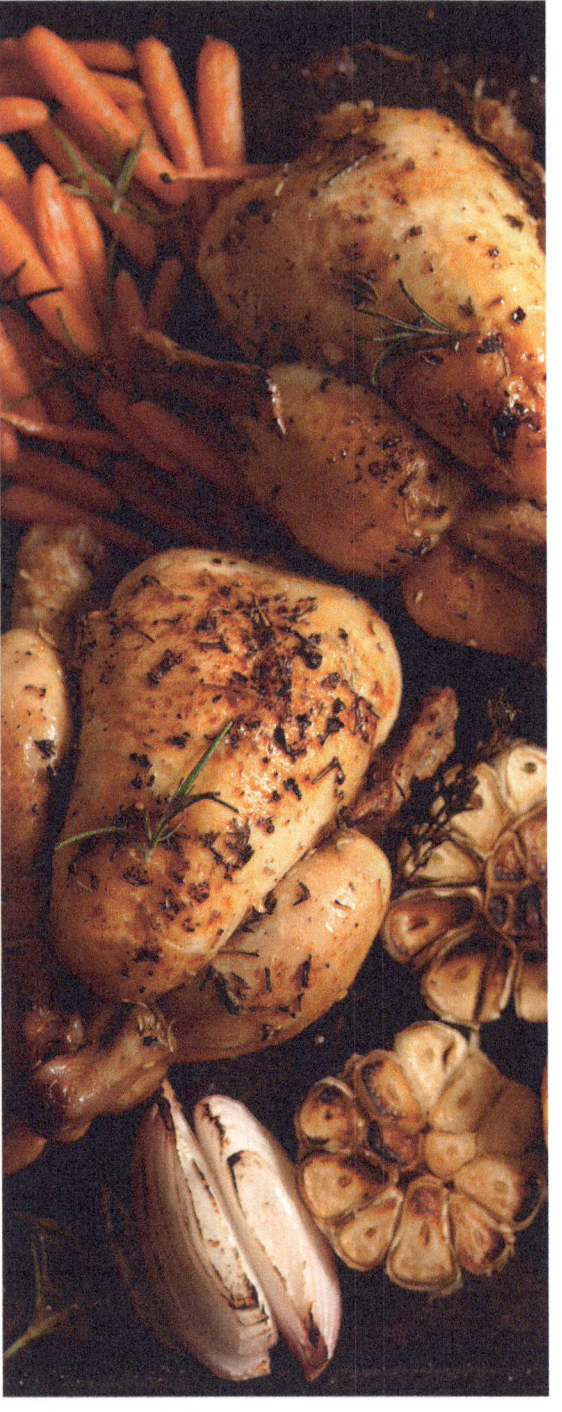

Ingredients:
- 1 lb. boneless, skinless chicken breast
- 2 carrots, diced
- 1 red onion, diced
- 1 head garlic, cloves peeled
- 1/4 cup olive oil
- salt and pepper to taste

Instructions:
1. Preheat oven to 375 degrees F.
2. In a large bowl, mix together chicken, carrots, red onion, garlic cloves, olive oil, salt and pepper until well combined.
3. Spread mixture in an even layer on a baking sheet lined with foil or parchment paper.
4. Bake for 25-30 minutes or until chicken is cooked through and vegetables are tender. Serve immediately!

Serving size: 1 chicken breast with 1/2 cup roasted vegetables
Calories: 560

SALMON WITH QUINOA AND ROASTED VEGETABLES

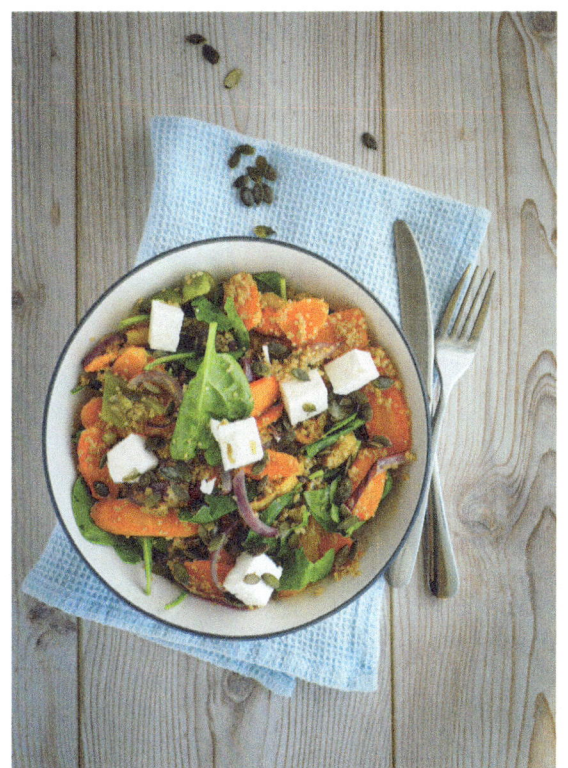

Ingredients:
- 1 lb. salmon
- 1 cup quinoa, cooked according to package instructions
- 2 carrots, diced
- 1 red onion, diced
- 1 head garlic, cloves peeled
- 1/4 cup olive oil
- salt and pepper to taste

Instructions:
1. Preheat oven to 375 degrees F.
2. In a large bowl, mix together cooked quinoa, carrots, red onion, garlic cloves, olive oil, salt and pepper until well combined.
3. Spread mixture in an even layer on a baking sheet lined with foil or parchment paper. Place salmon fillets on top of quinoa mixture.
4. Bake for 25-30 minutes or until salmon is cooked through and vegetables are tender. Serve immediately!

Serving size: 1 salmon fillet with 1/2 cup quinoa and roasted vegetables
Calories: 570

CHICKEN CURRY WITH COCONUT MILK AND RICE

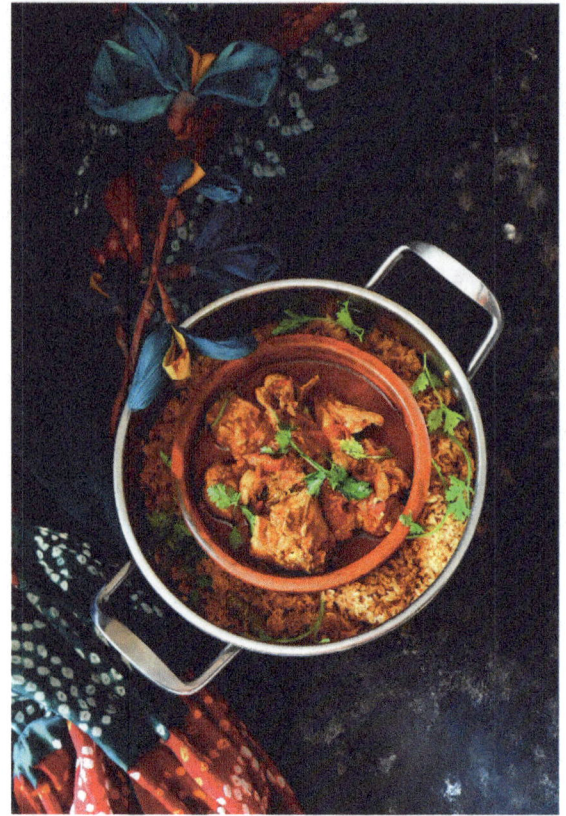

Ingredients:
- 1 lb. boneless, skinless chicken breast, cut into cubes
- 1 can (13.5 oz.) coconut milk
- 1 onion, diced
- 3 cloves garlic, minced
- 1 tbsp. freshly grated ginger
- 1 tbsp. red curry paste
- 1 tsp. ground turmeric
- 1/2 tsp. ground cumin
- salt and pepper to taste
- 1 cup cooked rice

Instructions:
1. In a large pot or Dutch oven, heat coconut milk over medium heat.
2. Add onions, garlic, ginger, red curry paste, turmeric, cumin, salt and pepper and cook until fragrant.
3. Stir in chicken cubes and cook until chicken is cooked through.
4. Season with additional salt and pepper to taste. Serve curry over cooked rice.

Serving size: 1 cup chicken curry with 1/2 cup cooked rice
Calories: 580

BEEF STEW WITH POTATOES AND CARROTS

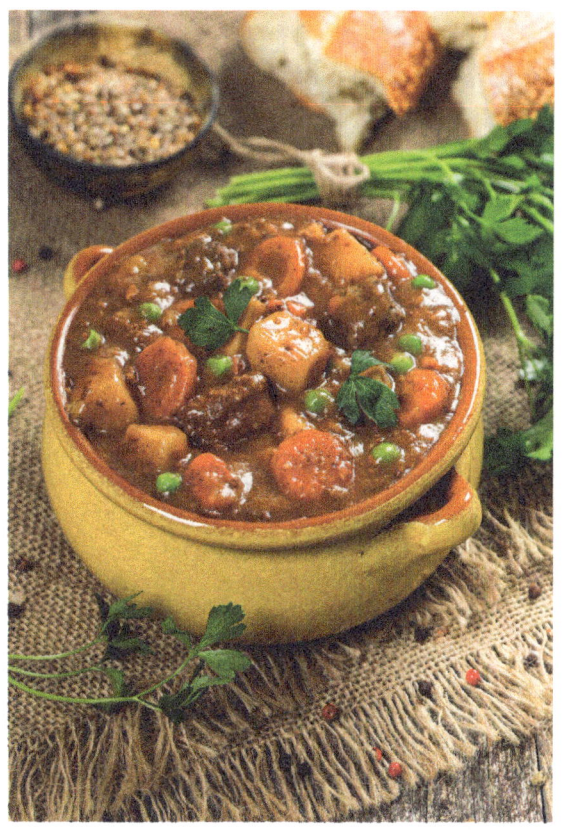

Ingredients:
- 1 lb. beef stew meat
- 2 cups beef broth
- 1 can (14.5 oz.) diced tomatoes
- 1 onion, diced
- 3 cloves garlic, minced
- 2 carrots, diced
- 2 potatoes, diced
- 1 tbsp. tomato paste
- 1 tsp. dried thyme leave
- 1/4 cup all-purpose flour
- salt and pepper to taste

Instructions:
1. In a large pot or Dutch oven, heat beef broth over medium heat.
2. Add onions, garlic, and carrots and cook until softened.
3. Stir in diced tomatoes, tomato paste, thyme leaves, and salt and pepper to taste.
4. Add beef stew meat and cook until browned.
5. Stir in potatoes and cook until tender.
6. If stew is too thin, whisk flour into 1/4 cup of cold water and stir into stew. Cook until thickened. Serve immediately!

Serving size: 1 cup beef stew with 1/2 cup vegetables
Calories: 590

TURKEY CHILI

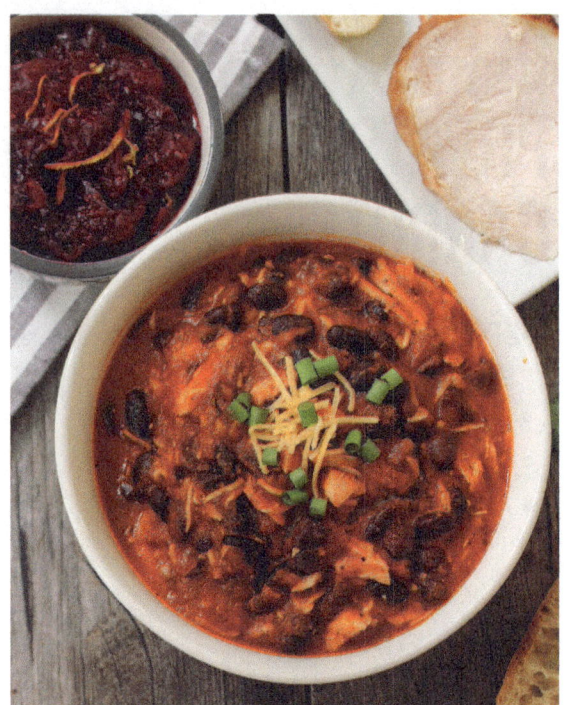

Ingredients:
- 1 lb. ground turkey
- 1 can (15 oz.) kidney beans, drained and rinsed
- 1 can (15 oz.) black beans, drained and rinsed
- 1 can (14.5 oz.) diced tomatoes
- 1 onion, diced
- 3 cloves garlic, minced
- 1 green bell pepper, diced
- 1 tsp. chili powder
- 1 tsp. cumin
- salt and pepper to taste

Instructions:
1. In a large pot or Dutch oven, cook ground turkey over medium heat until browned.
2. Add onions, garlic, and bell pepper and cook until softened.
3. Stir in chili powder and cumin and cook for 1 minute.
4. Add diced tomatoes, kidney beans, black beans, salt and pepper to taste.
5. Bring to a simmer and cook for 10 minutes. Serve immediately!

Serving size: 1 cup turkey chili
Calories: 600

BAKED HAM WITH SWEET POTATO CASSEROLE AND GREEN BEANS

Ingredients:
- 1 lb. ham
- 1 can (29 oz.) pineapple chunks, drained
- 1/4 cup brown sugar
- 2 tbsp. cornstarch
- 1/2 tsp. ground cloves
- 1 sweet potato, peeled and cut into cubes
- 1/4 cup melted butter
- 1/4 cup maple syrup
- 1/2 tsp. salt
- 1/4 tsp. black pepper
- 2 cups green beans

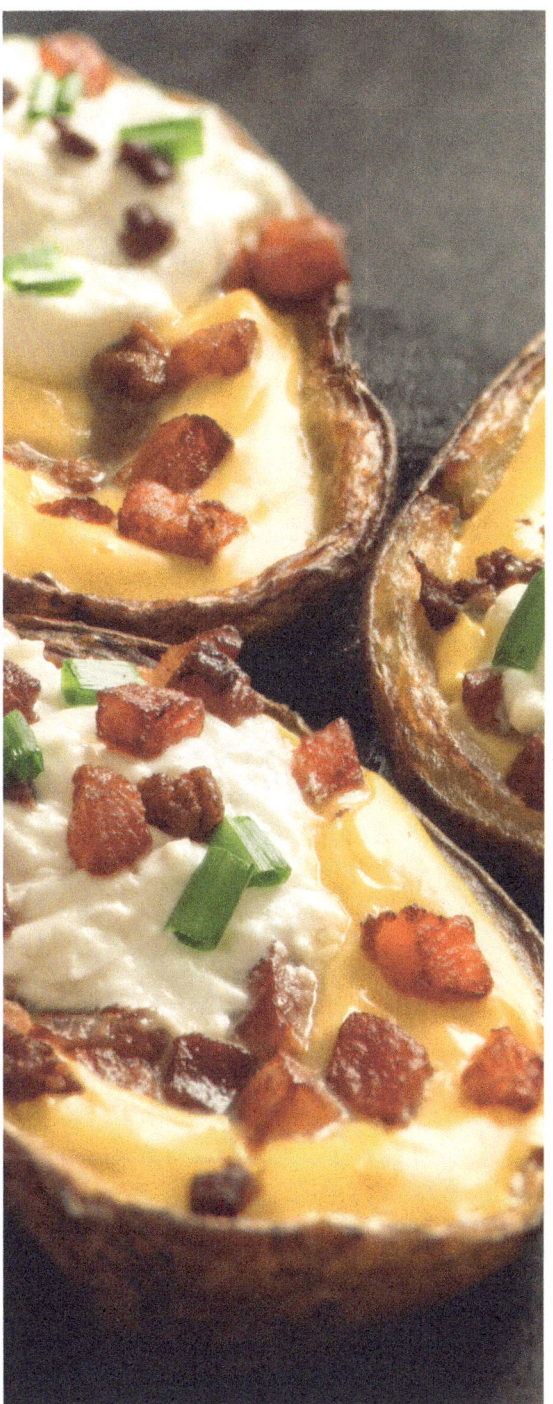

Instructions:
1. Preheat oven to 350 degrees F.
2. In a small saucepan, mix together pineapple chunks, brown sugar, cornstarch and ground cloves. Cook over medium heat until mixture thickens and bubbly. Set aside.
3. In a large casserole dish, place ham. Pour pineapple mixture over top of ham.
4. In a medium bowl, mix together sweet potato cubes, melted butter, maple syrup, salt and pepper. Pour over top of ham and pineapple mixture.
5. Cover with foil and bake for 1 hour. Remove foil and bake for an additional 30 minutes or until sweet potatoes are tender.
6. During the last 30 minutes of baking time, cook green beans in boiling water for 3-5 minutes or until tender. Drain and serve with ham and sweet potato casserole.

Serving size: 1/2 cup ham with 1/2 cup sweet potato casserole and 1/2 cup green beans
Calories: 610

SHEPHERD'S PIE

Ingredients:
- 1 lb. ground lamb
- 1 onion, diced
- 3 cloves garlic, minced
- 1 carrot, peeled and diced
- 1 celery stalk, diced
- 1/4 cup all-purpose flour
- 2 cups beef broth
- 1 tsp. dried thyme leaves
- 1/2 cup frozen peas
- 2 large potatoes, peeled and cut into cubes
- 1/4 cup milk
- salt and pepper to taste

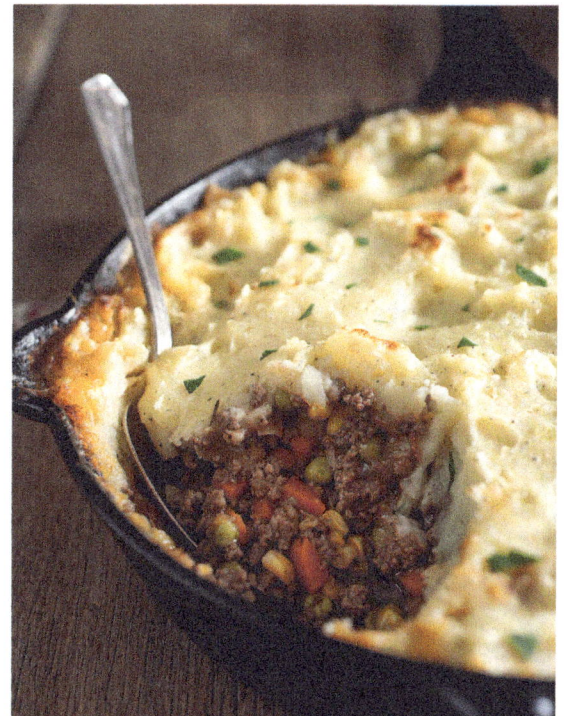

Instructions:
1. Preheat oven to 350 degrees F.
2. In a large pot or Dutch oven, cook ground lamb over medium heat until browned.
3. Add onions, garlic, carrots and celery and cook until softened.
4. Stir in flour and cook for 1 minute.
5. Add beef broth and thyme leaves and bring to a simmer. Cook for 10 minutes.
6. Stir in frozen peas and remove from heat.
7. In a large pot, boil potatoes until tender. Drain and mash with milk, salt and pepper to taste.
8. Spread mashed potatoes over top of lamb mixture in Dutch oven. Bake for 20-30 minutes or until potatoes are golden brown. Serve immediately!

Serving size: 1 cup shepherd's pie
Calories: 620

SALMON CAKES WITH ROASTED VEGETABLES

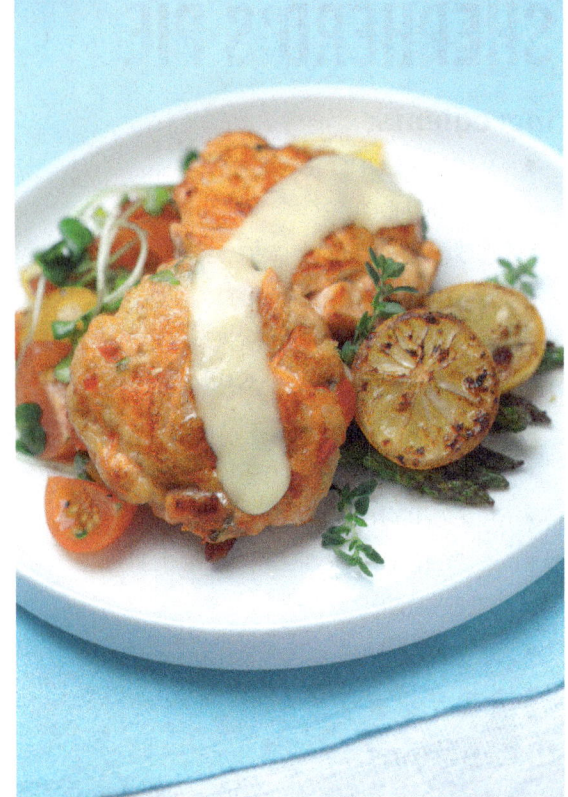

Ingredients:
- 1 lb. skinless, boneless salmon
- 1 egg, beaten
- 1/4 cup bread crumbs
- 1/4 cup diced onion
- 1 tbsp. minced fresh parsley
- 1 tsp. dried dill weed
- salt and pepper to taste
- 1/4 cup olive oil, divided
- 2 cups broccoli florets
- 1 red bell pepper, cut into chunks
- 1 yellow squash, sliced

Instructions:
1. Preheat oven to 400 degrees F.
2. In a large bowl, mix together salmon, egg, bread crumbs, onion, parsley, dill weed, salt and pepper to taste. Form into small cakes.
3. In a large skillet over medium heat, heat 2 tablespoons olive oil. Add salmon cakes and cook for 4 minutes per side or until golden brown. Remove from heat and set aside.
4. In a large roasting pan, toss together broccoli florets, bell pepper, yellow squash and remaining olive oil. Roast in preheated oven for 20 minutes or until vegetables are tender. Serve immediately with salmon cakes.

Serving size: 2 salmon cakes with 1/2 cup roasted vegetables
Calories: 630

BEEF STROGANOFF

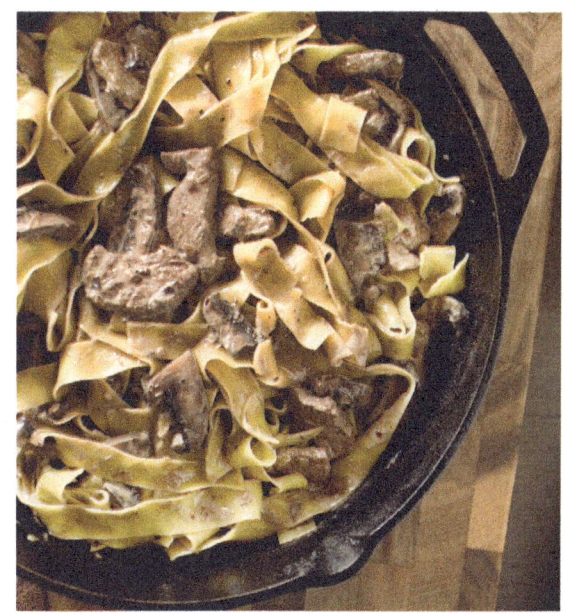

Ingredients:
- 1 lb. beef tenderloin, cut into cubes
- salt and pepper to taste
- 1 tbsp. olive oil
- 1 onion, diced
- 8 oz. mushrooms, sliced
- 3 cloves garlic, minced
- 1/4 cup gluten-free flour
- 1 cup beef broth
- 1/4 cup sour cream

Instructions:
1. Season beef cubes with salt and pepper. Heat olive oil in a large pot or Dutch oven over medium heat. Add beef and cook until browned on all sides. Remove from pot and set aside.
2. Add onion, mushrooms and garlic to the pot and cook until softened.
3. Stir in flour and cook for 1 minute.
4. Add beef broth and bring to a simmer, stirring constantly.
5. Return beef to the pot and stir in sour cream. Cook until heated through. Serve immediately!

Serving size: 1/2 cup beef stroganoff
Calories: 640

MEATLOAF WITH MASHED POTATOES AND CARROTS

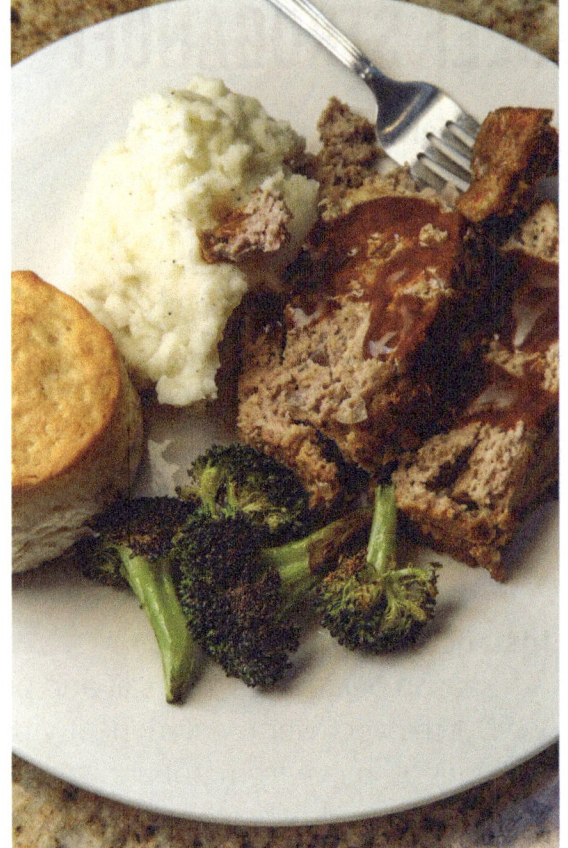

Ingredients:
- 1 lb. ground beef
- 1/2 cup bread crumbs
- 1 onion, diced
- 1 egg, beaten
- 1/4 cup ketchup
- 1 tsp. mustard
- salt and pepper to taste
- 3 carrots, peeled and cut into chunks
- 2 potatoes, peeled and cut into cubes
- 1/4 cup milk

Instructions:
1. Preheat oven to 350 degrees F.
2. In a large bowl, mix together ground beef, bread crumbs, onion, egg, ketchup, mustard, salt and pepper to taste. Form into a loaf shape and place in a baking dish.
3. Bake for 1 hour or until cooked through.
4. Meanwhile, place carrots and potatoes in a large pot of boiling water. Cook until tender. Drain and mash with milk, salt and pepper to taste.
5. Serve meatloaf with mashed potatoes and carrots.

Serving size: 1/2 cup meatloaf with 1/4 cup mashed potatoes and 1 carrot
Calories: 650

ROASTED TURKEY BREAST WITH STUFFING AND GREEN BEANS

Ingredients:
- 1 (4 lb.) turkey breast
- salt and pepper to taste
- 1 tbsp. olive oil
- 1 onion, diced
- 1 celery stalk, diced
- 1/2 cup bread crumbs
- 1/4 cup chopped fresh parsley
- 1 tsp. sage leaves
- 1/4 cup chicken broth
- 1 (16 oz.) package frozen green beans

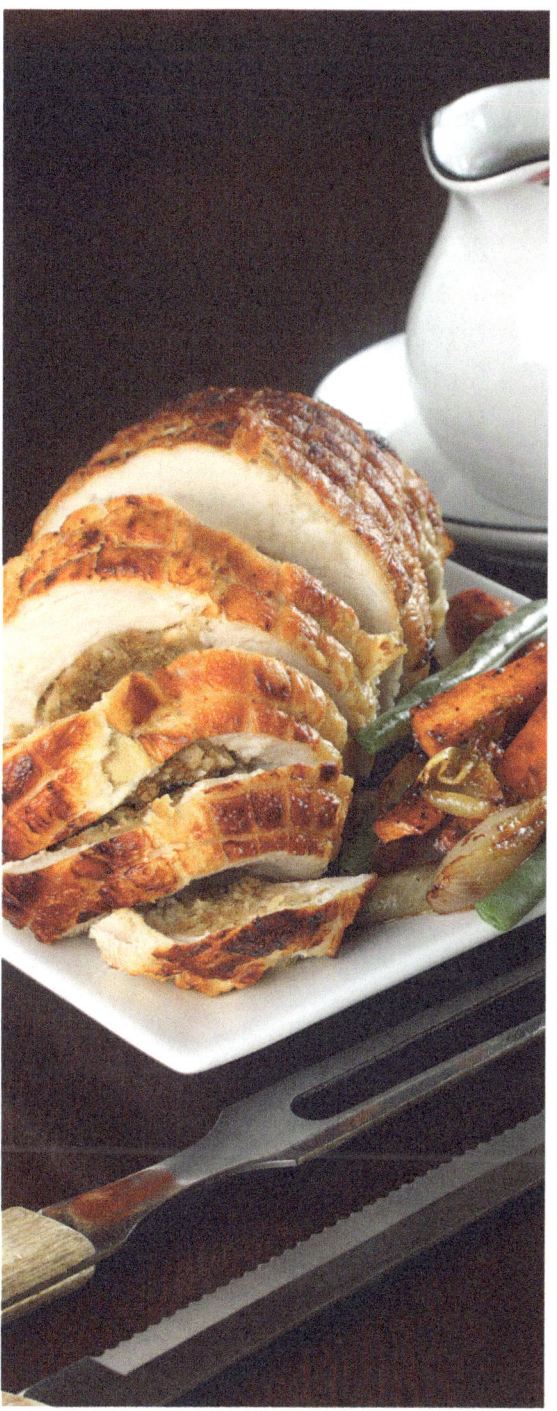

Instructions:
1. Preheat oven to 325 degrees F.
2. Season turkey breast with salt and pepper. Heat olive oil in a large skillet over medium heat. Add turkey and cook until browned on all sides. Remove from heat and set aside.
3. Add onion and celery to the skillet and cook until softened.
4. In a large bowl, mix together bread crumbs, parsley, sage leaves and chicken broth.
5. Stuff turkey breast with bread crumb mixture and place in a roasting pan. Bake for 2-3 hours or until cooked through.
6. About 30 minutes before turkey is done, cook green beans according to package instructions. Serve immediately with turkey.

Serving size: 1/2 cup roasted turkey with 1/4 cup stuffing and 1/2 cup green beans
Calories: 660

ROASTED PORK LOIN WITH SWEET POTATOES AND APPLES

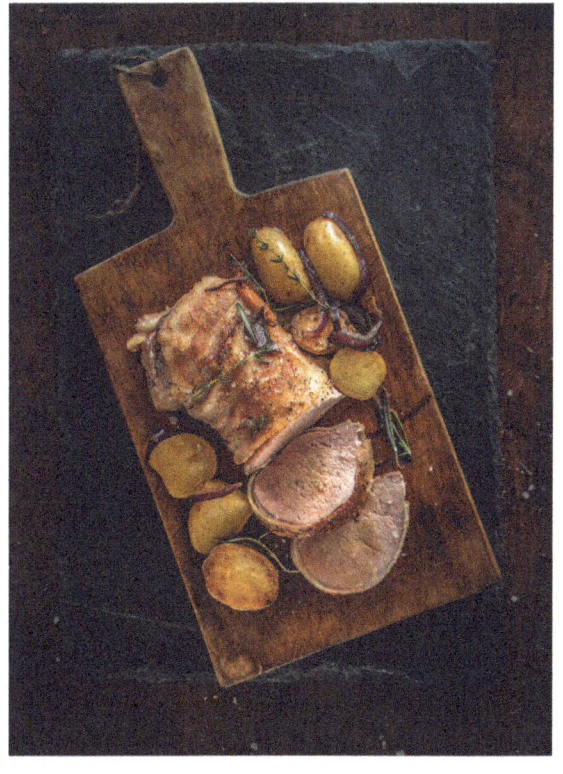

Ingredients:
- 1 (2 lb.) pork loin
- salt and pepper to taste
- 1 tbsp. olive oil
- 3 sweet potatoes, peeled and cut into chunks
- 2 apples, peeled and cut into chunks
- 1/4 cup apple cider

Instructions:
1. Preheat oven to 325 degrees F.
2. Season pork loin with salt and pepper. Heat olive oil in a large skillet over medium heat. Add pork and cook until browned on all sides. Remove from heat and set aside.
3. In a large roasting pan, mix together sweet potatoes, apples and apple cider. Place pork loin in the center of the pan.
4. Bake for 2-3 hours or until cooked through. Let rest for 10 minutes before slicing and serving.

Serving size: 1/2 cup roasted pork with 1/2 cup sweet potatoes and 1/2 apple
Calories: 670

VEGETABLE LASAGNA

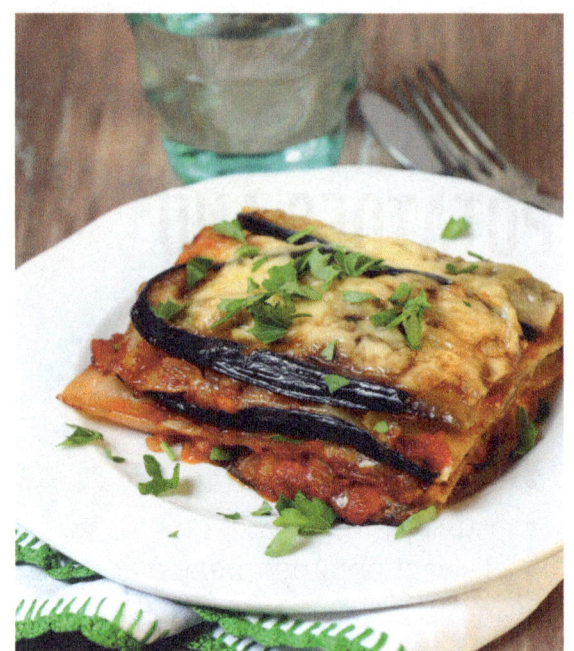

Ingredients:
- 1 (16 oz.) package lasagna noodles
- 1 (24 oz.) jar marinara sauce
- 1 (15 oz.) container ricotta cheese
- 1 egg, beaten
- 1/4 cup grated Parmesan cheese
- 2 cloves garlic, minced
- salt and pepper to taste
- 2 zucchini, thinly sliced lengthwise
- 1 (10 oz.) package frozen spinach, thawed and drained
- 1 cup shredded mozzarella cheese

Instructions:
1. Preheat oven to 375 degrees F.
2. In a large pot of boiling water, cook lasagna noodles according to package instructions. Drain and set aside.
3. In a medium bowl, mix together marinara sauce, ricotta cheese, egg, Parmesan cheese, garlic, salt and pepper to taste.
4. Spread 1/2 cup of the sauce mixture over the bottom of a 9x13 inch baking dish. Layer with 3 noodles, 1/2 of the zucchini slices, 1/2 of the spinach and 1/3 of the mozzarella cheese. Repeat layers.
5. Cover with aluminum foil and bake for 30 minutes. Remove from oven and let rest for 10 minutes before serving.

Serving size: 1 piece lasagna
Calories: 680

BEEF STEW

Ingredients:
- 2 lbs. beef stew meat
- salt and pepper to taste
- 1 tbsp. olive oil
- 4 carrots, peeled and cut into chunks
- 2 potatoes, peeled and cut into chunks
- 1 onion, diced
- 3 cloves garlic, minced
- 1 (14.5 oz.) can diced tomatoes
- 1 (10.75 oz.) can beef broth
- 1 bay leaf
- 1/4 tsp. thyme leaves

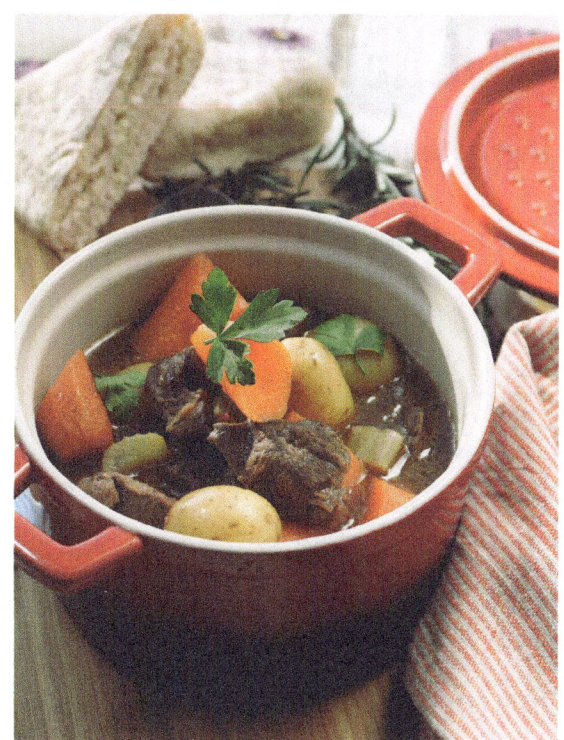

Instructions:
1. Season beef stew meat with salt and pepper. Heat olive oil in a large pot over medium heat. Add beef and cook until browned on all sides. Remove from heat and set aside.
2. Add carrots, potatoes, onion and garlic to the pot and cook until softened.
3. Stir in diced tomatoes, beef broth, bay leaf and thyme leaves. Add beef back into the pot.
4. Bring to a simmer and cook for 2-3 hours or until beef is cooked through. Remove bay leaf before serving.

Serving size: 1 cup beef stew
Calories: 690

CHICKEN POT PIE

Ingredients:
- 1 (9 inch) pie crust, store bought or homemade
- 1/4 cup butter
- 1/4 cup all-purpose flour
- 1/2 tsp. salt
- 1/4 tsp. black pepper
- 2 cups chicken broth
- 1/2 cup milk
- 2 cups cooked, shredded chicken
- 1 (10 oz.) package frozen mixed vegetables, thawed

Instructions:
1. Preheat oven to 375 degrees F.
2. In a large pot, melt butter over medium heat. Stir in flour, salt and pepper until smooth.
3. Add chicken broth and milk, and whisk until smooth.
4. Stir in chicken and vegetables. Pour into pie crust.
5. Bake for 45 minutes or until crust is golden brown and filling is bubbly.

Serving size: 1/8 of pie
Calories: 700

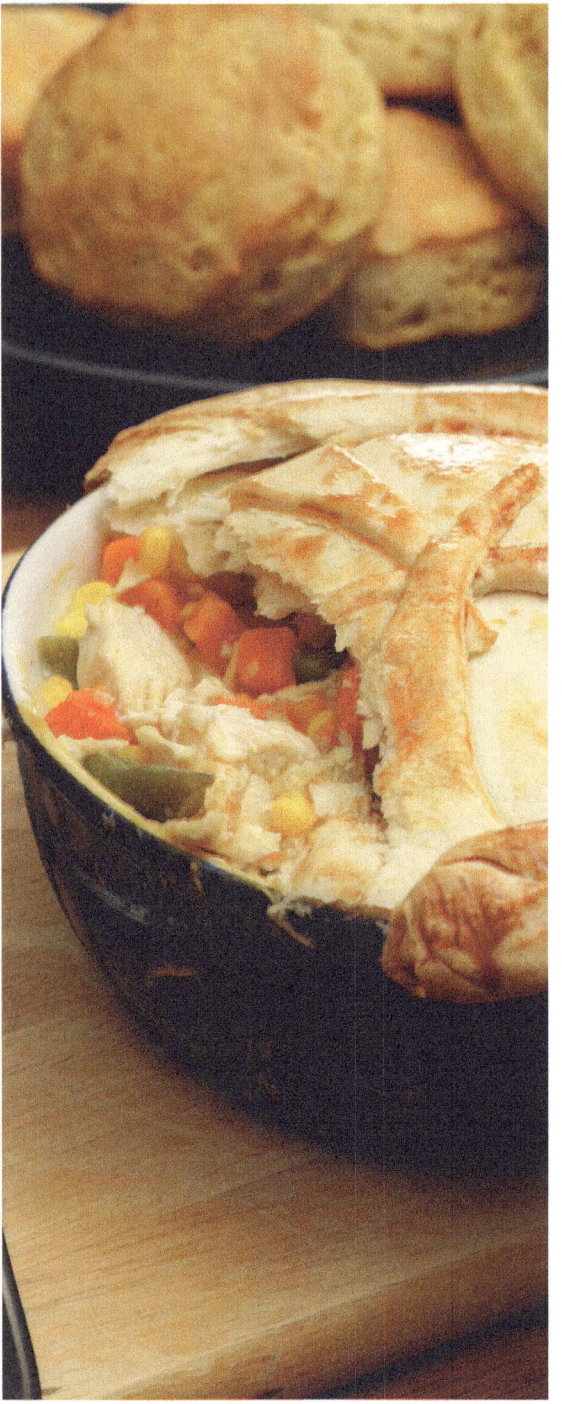

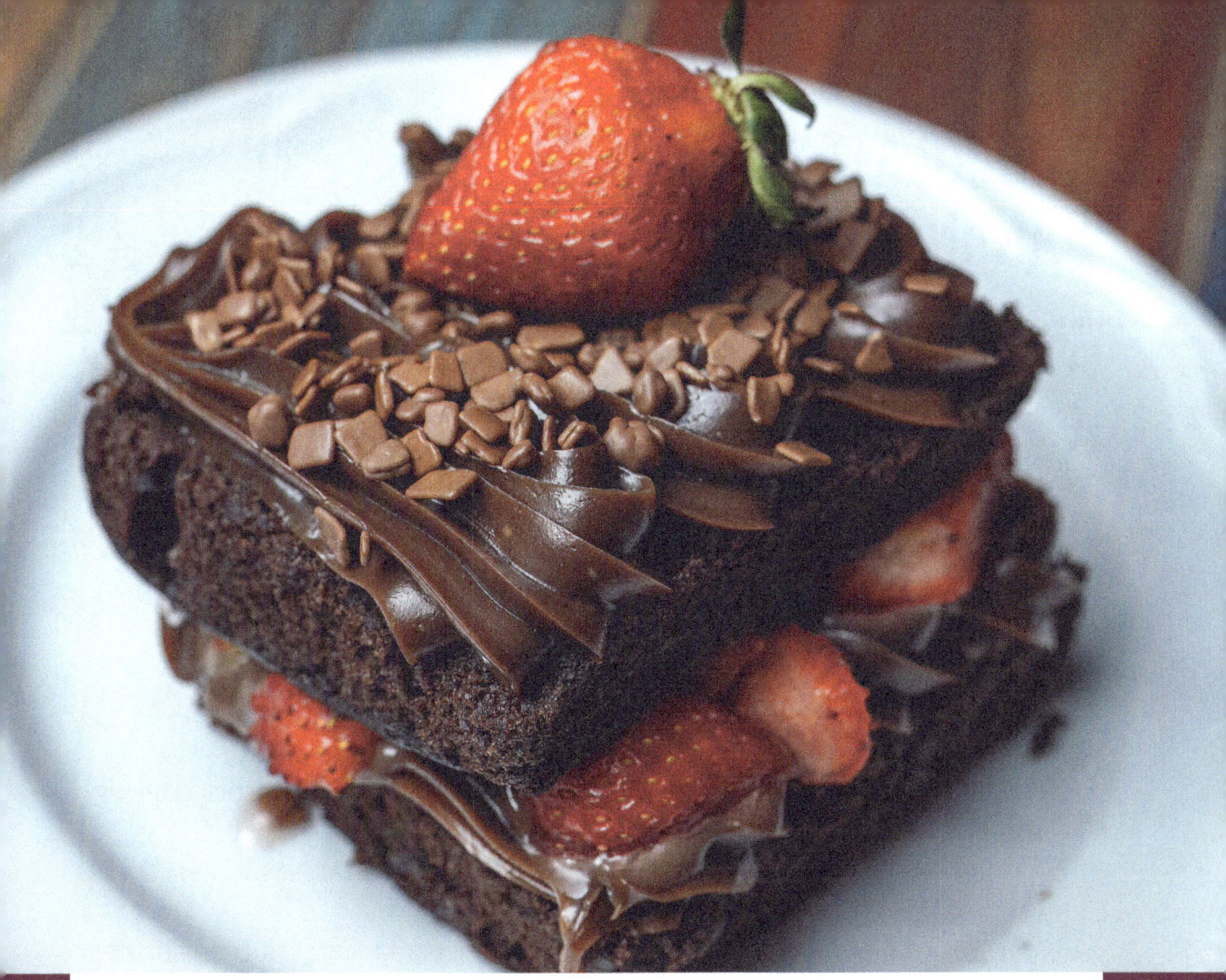

CHAPTER SIX: DESSERTS

CHOCOLATE CHIP BANANA BREAD

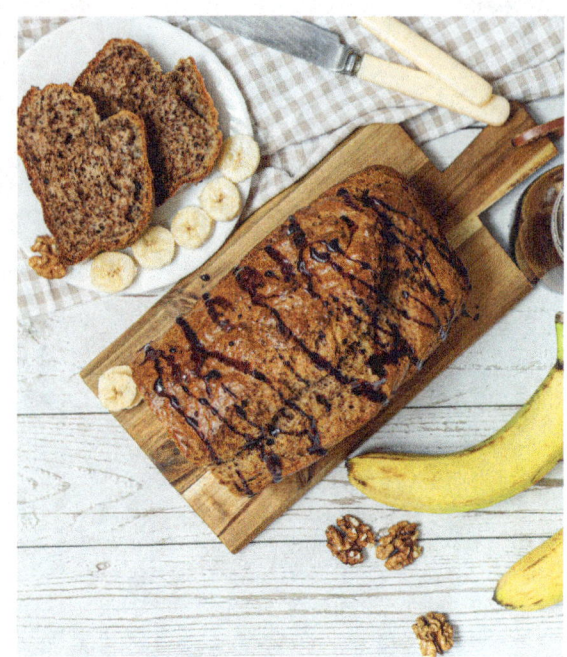

Ingredients:
- 3 ripe bananas, mashed
- 1/3 cup melted butter
- 1 cup sugar
- 1 egg, beaten
- 1 tsp. vanilla extract
- 2 cups gluten-free flour
- 1 tsp. baking soda
- 1/2 tsp. salt
- 1 cup chocolate chips

Instructions:
1. Preheat oven to 350 degrees F and spray a loaf pan with non-stick cooking spray.
2. In a large bowl, combine mashed bananas, melted butter, sugar, egg, and vanilla extract until well combined.
3. In a separate bowl, whisk together flour, baking soda, and salt then stir into wet ingredients until just combined (be careful not to overmix).
4. Gently fold in chocolate chips then pour batter into prepared loaf pan.
5. Bake for 50-60 minutes or until a toothpick inserted into the center comes out clean.
6. Allow bread to cool in the pan for 10 minutes before removing to a wire rack to cool completely.

Serving size: 1 slice
Calories: 290

BLUEBERRY CRISP

Ingredients:
- 6 cups fresh blueberries, divided
- 1/4 cup sugar
- 1 tbsp. cornstarch
- 1/2 tsp. grated lemon zest
- 1/4 tsp. ground cinnamon

Topping:
- 1 cup old-fashioned rolled oats
- 1/2 cup gluten-free flour
- 1/4 cup packed brown sugar
- 1/4 cup cold butter
- 1/2 tsp. ground cinnamon
- 1/4 tsp. ground ginger

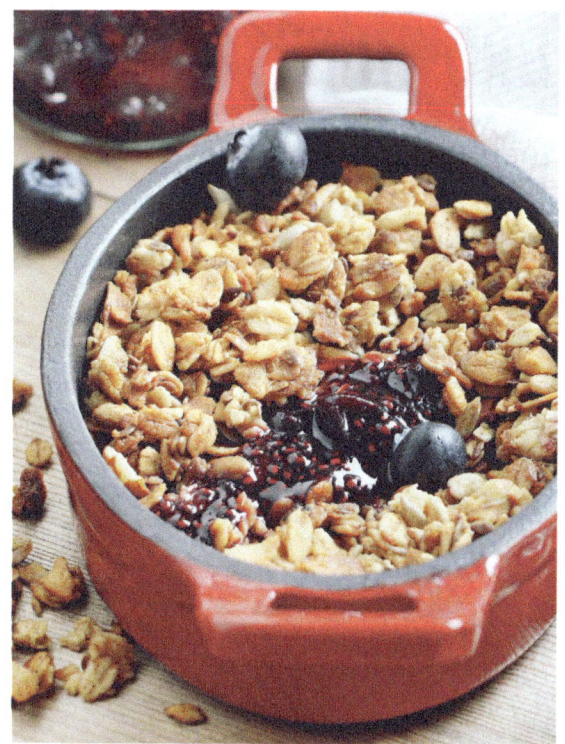

Instructions:
1. Preheat oven to 375 degrees F and spray an 8x8 inch baking dish with non-stick cooking spray.
2. In a large bowl, combine 3 cups blueberries, sugar, cornstarch, lemon zest, and cinnamon then pour into the prepared baking dish.
3. In the same bowl (no need to wash), combine oats, flour, brown sugar, butter, cinnamon and ginger then crumble over the top of the blueberry mixture.
4. Bake for 40-45 minutes or until topping is golden brown and filling is bubbly.
5. Remove from oven and let cool for 10-15 minutes before serving.

Serving size: 1/9 of crisp
Calories: 310

BROWNIES

Ingredients:
- 1/2 cup butter, melted
- 1 cup sugar
- 2 eggs
- 1 tsp. vanilla extract
- 1/3 cup unsweetened cocoa powder
- 1/2 cup gluten-free flour
- 1/4 tsp. baking powder
- 1/4 tsp. salt
- 1 cup chocolate chips

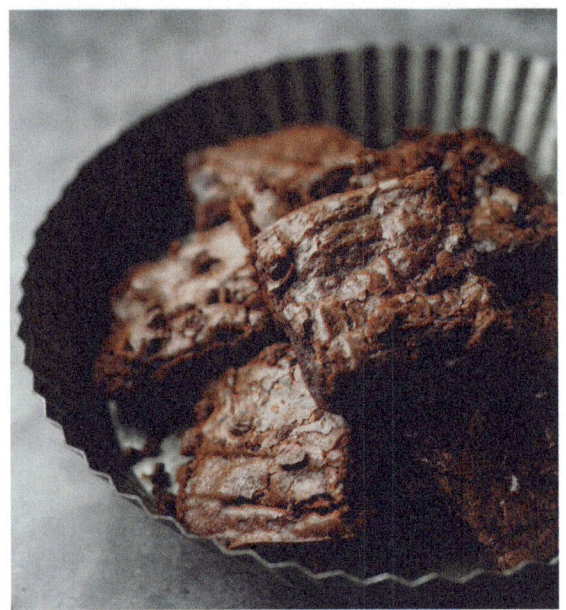

Instructions:
1. Preheat oven to 350 degrees F and spray an 8x8 inch baking dish with non-stick cooking spray.
2. In a large bowl, whisk together melted butter, sugar, eggs and vanilla extract until well combined.
3. Stir in cocoa powder, flour, baking powder and salt then fold in chocolate chips.
4. Pour batter into prepared pan and bake for 22-25 minutes or until a toothpick inserted into the center comes out with just a few moist crumbs attached.
5. Allow brownies to cool completely before cutting into squares.

Serving size: 1 brownie
Calories: 210

CHOCOLATE CHIP COOKIES

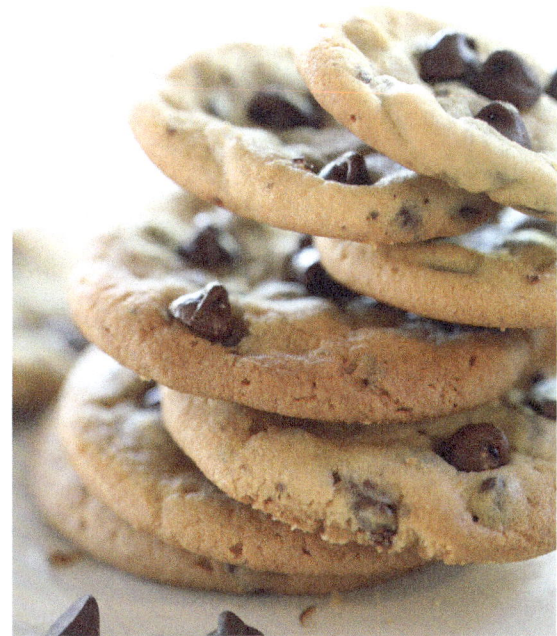

Ingredients:
- 2/3 cup butter, softened
- 1/2 cup sugar
- 1/2 cup packed brown sugar
- 1 tsp. vanilla extract
- 2 eggs
- 1-1/2 cups gluten-free flour
- 1 tsp. baking soda
- 1/2 tsp. salt
- 2 cups semisweet chocolate chips

Instructions:
1. Preheat oven to 350 degrees F and line a baking sheet with a silicone baking mat or parchment paper.
2. In a large bowl, cream together butter, sugar, brown sugar and vanilla extract until light and fluffy.
3. Beat in eggs one at a time then stir in flour, baking soda and salt until dough comes together.
4. Fold in chocolate chips then drop dough by rounded tablespoons onto the prepared baking sheet.
5. Bake for 9-11 minutes or until cookies are lightly golden brown and set. Allow cookies to cool on the baking sheet for a few minutes before transferring to a wire rack to cool completely.

Serving size: 1 cookie
Calories: 140

OATMEAL CHOCOLATE CHIP COOKIES

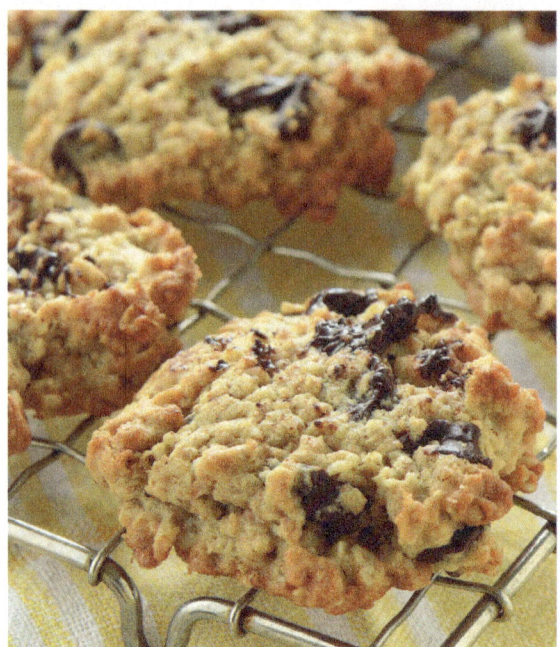

Ingredients:
- 1/2 cup butter, melted and cooled
- 1 cup packed brown sugar
- 1 egg, beaten
- 1 tsp. vanilla extract
- 1-1/4 cups gluten-free flour
- 1 tsp. baking soda
- 1/4 tsp. salt
- 3 cups quick-cooking oats
- 1 cup semisweet chocolate chips

Instructions:
1. Preheat oven to 350 degrees F and line a baking sheet with a silicone baking mat or parchment paper.
2. In a large bowl, whisk together melted butter, brown sugar, egg and vanilla extract until well combined.
3. Stir in flour, baking soda and salt then fold in oats and chocolate chips.
4. Drop dough by rounded tablespoons onto the prepared baking sheet.
5. Bake for 10-12 minutes or until cookies are lightly golden brown and set. Allow cookies to cool on the baking sheet for a few minutes before transferring to a wire rack to cool completely.

Serving size: 1 cookie
Calories: 190

PEANUT BUTTER COOKIES

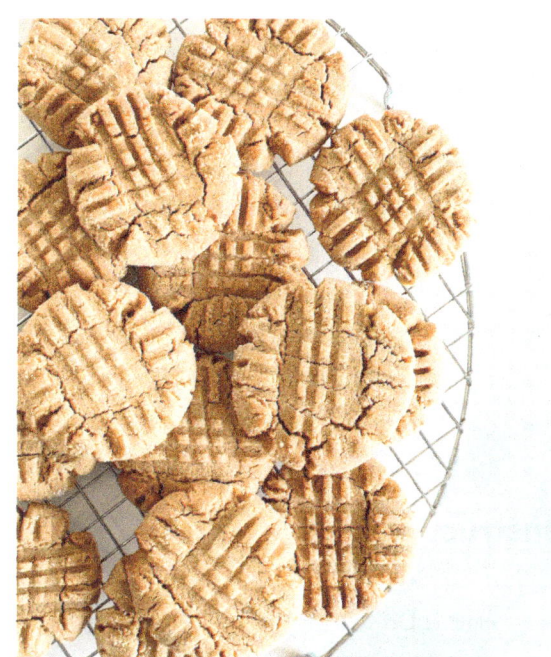

Ingredients:
- 1/2 cup butter, softened
- 1/2 cup sugar
- 1/2 cup packed brown sugar
- 1/2 cup creamy peanut butter
- 1 tsp. vanilla extract
- 1 egg
- 1-1/4 cups gluten-free flour
- 3/4 tsp. baking soda
- 1/2 tsp. salt

Instructions:
1. Preheat oven to 350 degrees F and line a baking sheet with a silicone baking mat or parchment paper.
2. In a large bowl, cream together butter, sugar, brown sugar, peanut butter and vanilla extract until light and fluffy.
3. Beat in egg then stir in flour, baking soda and salt until dough comes together.
4. Drop dough by rounded tablespoons onto the prepared baking sheet.
5. Bake for 9-11 minutes or until cookies are lightly golden brown and set. Allow cookies to cool on the baking sheet for a few minutes before transferring to a wire rack to cool completely.

Serving size: 1 cookie
Calories: 150

SUGAR COOKIES

Ingredients:
- 1/2 cup butter, softened
- 1/2 cup sugar
- 1 egg
- 1 tsp. vanilla extract
- 1-1/4 cups gluten-free flour
- 3/4 tsp. baking powder
- 1/4 tsp. salt

Instructions:
1. Preheat oven to 350 degrees F and line a baking sheet with a silicone baking mat or parchment paper.
2. In a large bowl, cream together butter and sugar until light and fluffy.
3. Beat in egg and vanilla extract then stir in flour, baking powder and salt until dough comes together.
4. Drop dough by rounded tablespoons onto the prepared baking sheet.
5. Bake for 9-11 minutes or until cookies are lightly golden brown and set. Allow cookies to cool on the baking sheet for a few minutes before transferring to a wire rack to cool completely.

Serving size: 1 cookie
Calories: 130

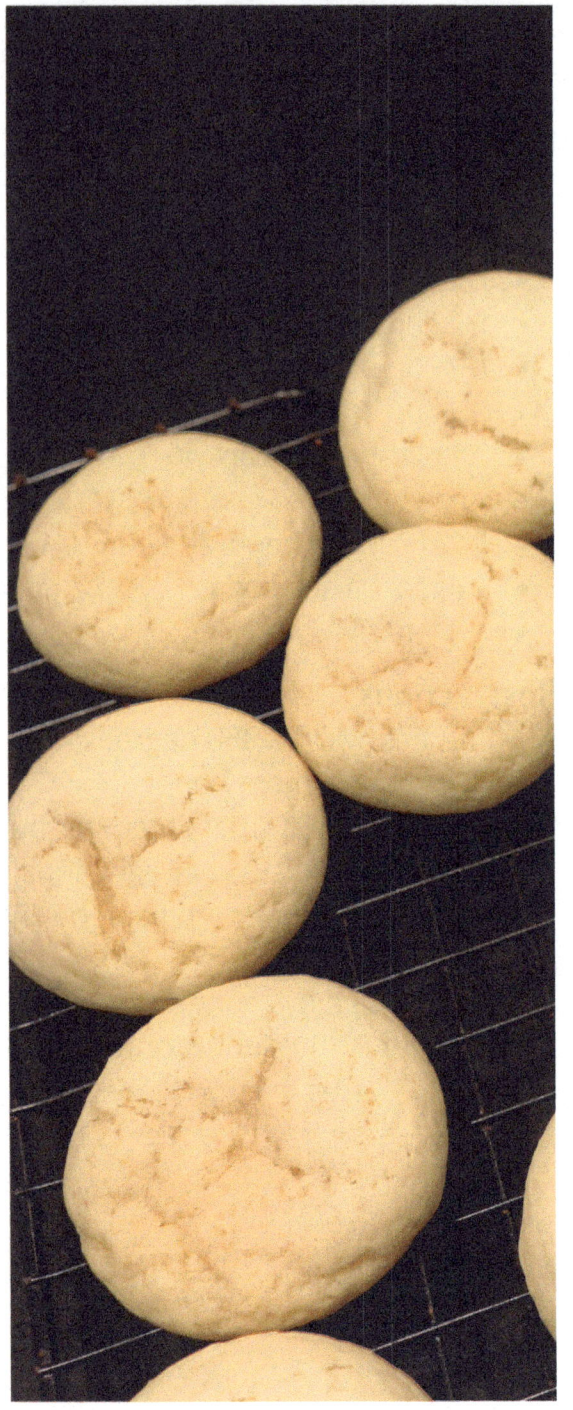

OREO CHEESECAKE BITES

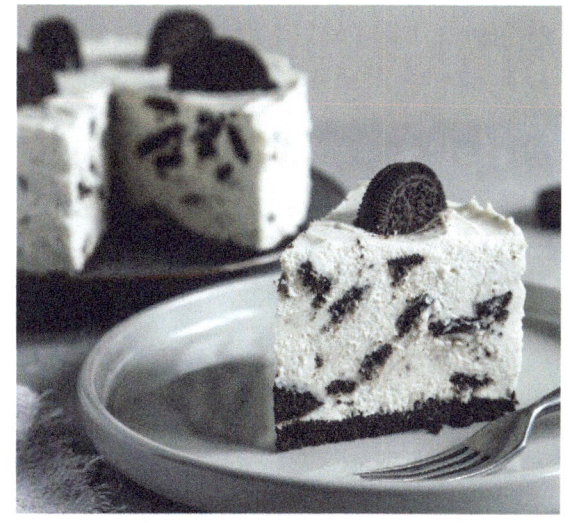

Ingredients:
- 24 Oreos, divided
- 4 oz. cream cheese, softened
- 1/4 cup sugar
- 1 tsp. vanilla extract
- 1 (8 oz.) package refrigerated crescent rolls

Instructions:
1. Preheat oven to 375 degrees F and line a baking sheet with parchment paper.
2. Place 12 Oreos in a food processor and pulse until finely crushed then set aside.
3. In a medium bowl, cream together cream cheese, sugar and vanilla extract until smooth.
4. Unroll crescent dough and separate into 8 triangles. Place a heaping tablespoon of the cream cheese mixture in the center of each triangle then top with 3-4 crushed Oreos.
5. Roll up each triangle, starting at the wide end, and place on the prepared baking sheet.
6. Bake for 11-13 minutes or until golden brown. Allow to cool for 5 minutes before serving.

Serving size: 2 bites
Calories: 190

STRAWBERRY SHORTCAKE

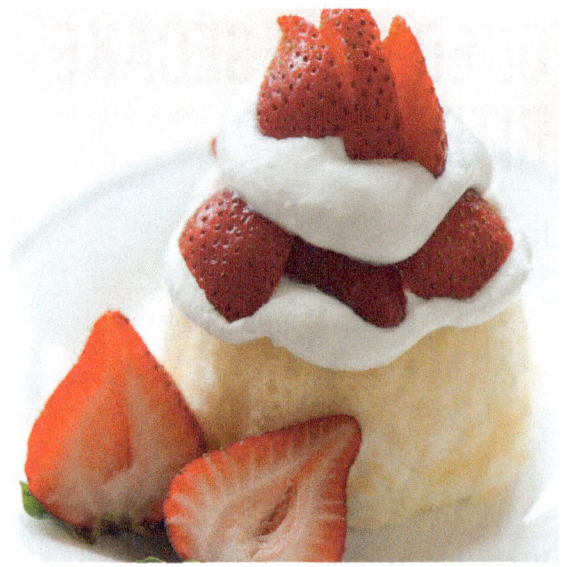

Ingredients:
- 1 (8 oz.) package refrigerated shortcake biscuits
- 1/2 cup sugar, divided
- 1 tsp. vanilla extract
- 1 lb. fresh strawberries, hulled and sliced
- 1 cup heavy cream

Instructions:
1. Preheat oven to 350 degrees F and line a baking sheet with parchment paper.
2. In a small bowl, whisk together 1/4 cup sugar, vanilla extract and heavy cream until well combined. Set aside.
3. Place biscuits on the prepared baking sheet and bake for 10-12 minutes or until golden brown. Allow to cool for 5 minutes then split each biscuit in half horizontally.
4. In a medium bowl, toss strawberries with remaining sugar until coated then let sit for 5 minutes to allow juices to release.
5. To assemble, place the bottom half of each biscuit on a plate then top with strawberries and a dollop of the cream mixture. Place the top half of the biscuit on top and serve immediately.

Serving size: 1 biscuit
Calories: 250

CHOCOLATE COVERED STRAWBERRIES

Ingredients:
- 1 pound strawberries
- 1 (12-ounce) package semi-sweet chocolate chips
- 1 tablespoon coconut oil

Instructions:
1. Line a baking sheet with parchment paper.
2. Wash strawberries then pat dry with a paper towel.
3. In a small saucepan, melt chocolate chips and coconut oil over low heat, stirring frequently until smooth.
4. Dip each strawberry into the chocolate mixture then place on the prepared baking sheet. Refrigerate for at least 30 minutes or until chocolate is set. Serve chilled.

Serving size: 1 strawberry
Calories: 50

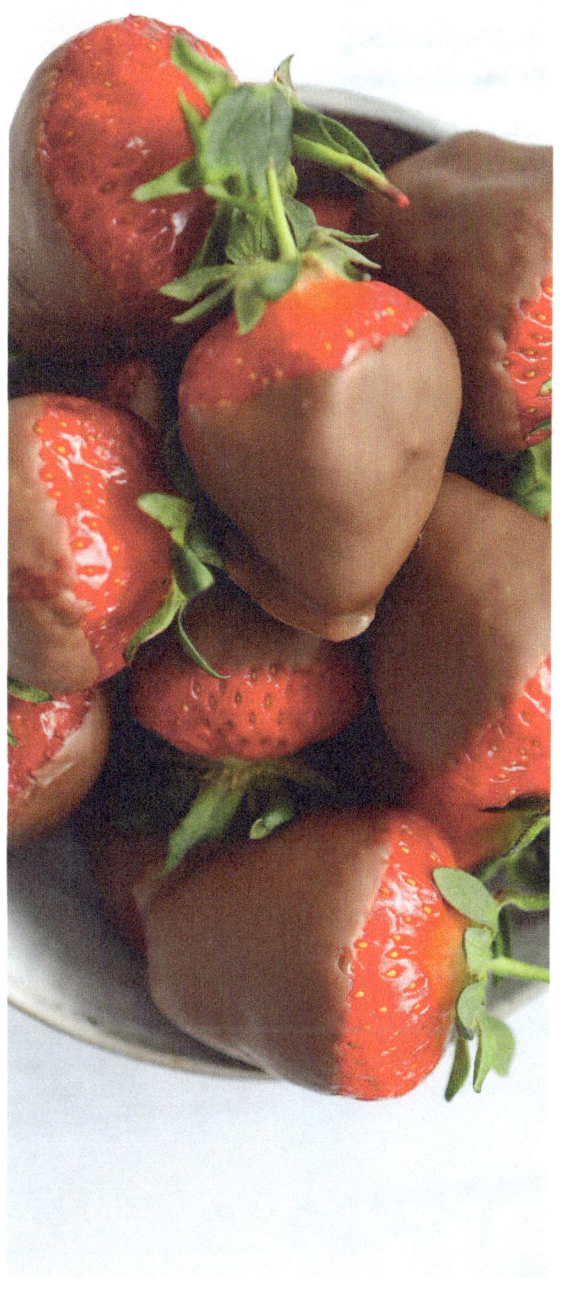

PEACH COBBLER

Ingredients:

Filling:
- 6-7 peaches, peeled and sliced
- 3/4 cup sugar
- 1/4 cup cornstarch
- 1 tsp. cinnamon
- 1/4 tsp. nutmeg
- Juice of 1 lemon

Topping:
- 1 cup gluten-free flour
- 3/4 cup sugar
- 1 tsp. baking powder
- 1/2 tsp. salt
- 6 tbsp. cold butter, cut into small pieces

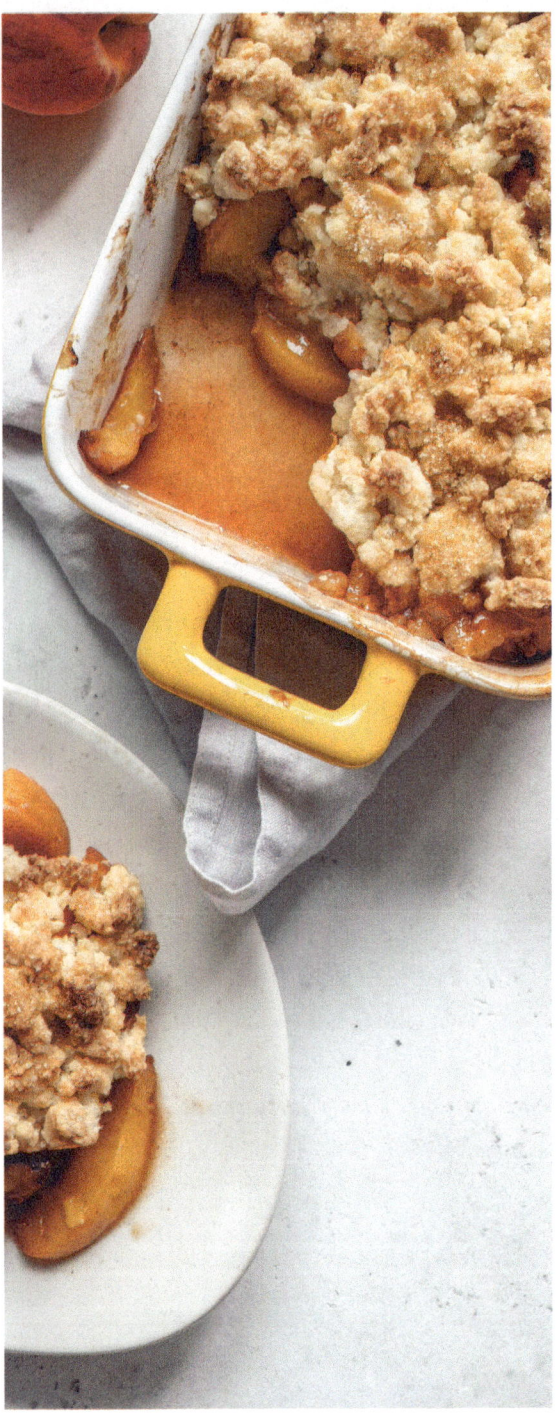

Instructions:
1. Preheat oven to 375 degrees F and coat a 9x13 inch baking dish with cooking spray.
2. To make the filling, add peaches, sugar, cornstarch, cinnamon, nutmeg and lemon juice to a large bowl then stir until evenly mixed. Pour mixture into the prepared baking dish and set aside.
3. To make the topping, add flour, sugar, baking powder and salt to a medium bowl then whisk until well combined. Cut in butter with a pastry blender or two knives until the mixture resembles coarse crumbs. Sprinkle evenly over the peach filling.
4. Bake for 45-50 minutes or until the top is golden brown and the filling is bubbly. Allow to cool for 10 minutes before serving warm with ice cream, if desired.

Serving size: 1/9 of recipe
Calories: 400

VANILLA PUDDING

Ingredients:
- 1/2 cup sugar
- 1/3 cup cornstarch
- 1/4 tsp. salt
- 3 cups milk (dairy or non-dairy)
- 1 vanilla bean, split lengthwise
- 3 egg yolks
- 2 tbsp. butter

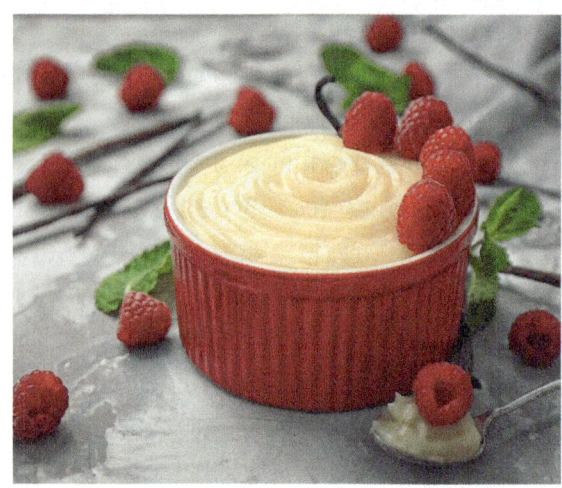

Instructions:
1. In a medium saucepan, whisk together sugar, cornstarch and salt then set aside.
2. Add milk to a small saucepan then heat over medium heat until just simmering. Slowly pour into the sugar mixture, whisking constantly until well combined.
3. Scrape seeds from vanilla bean into the milk mixture then add the bean pod. Stir until well combined then return to the heat and cook, stirring constantly, until mixture comes to a boil.
4. Remove from heat then slowly whisk in egg yolks until well combined.
5. Return to heat and cook, stirring constantly, until mixture comes to a boil. Remove from heat then whisk in butter until melted.
6. Pour pudding into a large bowl then press plastic wrap directly onto the surface of the pudding to prevent a skin from forming. Allow to cool for 1 hour then refrigerate for at least 2 hours or overnight. Serve chilled.

Serving size: 1/2 cup
Calories: 210

CRÈME BRULEE

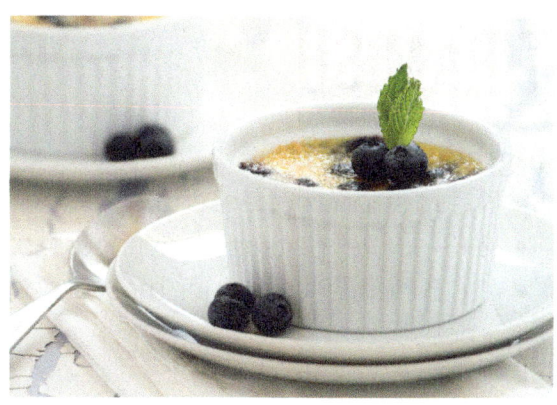

Ingredients:
- 2 cups heavy cream
- 1/2 cup sugar, divided
- 1 vanilla bean, split lengthwise
- 6 egg yolks
- 1/4 cup water

Instructions:
1. Preheat oven to 300 degrees F and place 8 (6-ounce) ramekins into a large baking dish.
2. Add cream, 1/4 cup sugar and vanilla bean to a medium saucepan then stir over low heat until sugar has dissolved and mixture is just simmering. Remove from heat and set aside.
3. In a medium bowl, whisk together egg yolks and remaining 1/4 cup sugar until well combined. Slowly pour in cream mixture, whisking constantly, until well combined.
4. Divide mixture evenly among the prepared ramekins then carefully pour enough hot water into the baking dish to come halfway up the sides of the ramekins.
5. Bake for 40-50 minutes or until custards are just set and slightly jiggly in the center. Remove from oven then allow to cool for 10 minutes.
6. Carefully remove ramekins from the water bath then refrigerate for at least 2 hours or overnight.
7. Just before serving, sprinkle 1 teaspoon sugar evenly over the top of each custard then use a kitchen torch to melt and caramelize the sugar. Allow to harden for 1-2 minutes before serving.

Serving size: 1 ramekin
Calories: 40

TIRAMISU

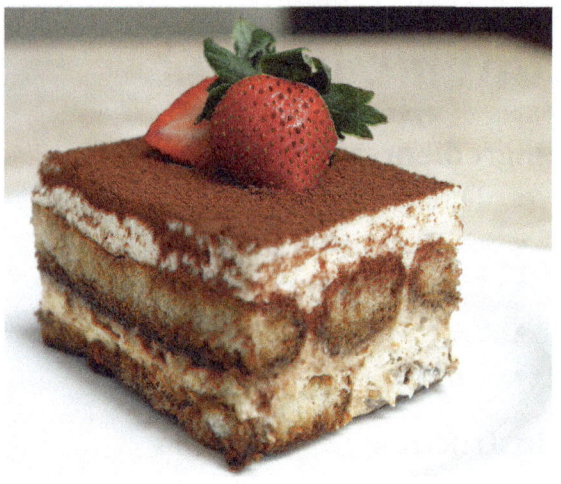

Ingredients:
- 1 cup strong coffee, cooled
- 1 (8-ounce) package ladyfingers
- 1 (15-ounce) container mascarpone cheese
- 1/2 cup sugar
- 1 teaspoon vanilla extract
- 1/4 cup cocoa powder

Instructions:
1. In a small bowl, combine coffee and 1 tablespoon sugar then stir until sugar has dissolved. Set aside.
2. In a large bowl, whisk together mascarpone, remaining sugar and vanilla until smooth.
3. Dip half of the ladyfingers into the coffee mixture then place in the bottom of an 8x8 inch baking dish. Spread half of the mascarpone mixture over the ladyfingers then sprinkle with half of the cocoa powder. Repeat layers with remaining ladyfingers, mascarpone mixture and cocoa powder.
4. Cover and refrigerate for at least 2 hours or overnight. Serve chilled.

Serving size: 1/9 of recipe
Calories: 380

FLAN

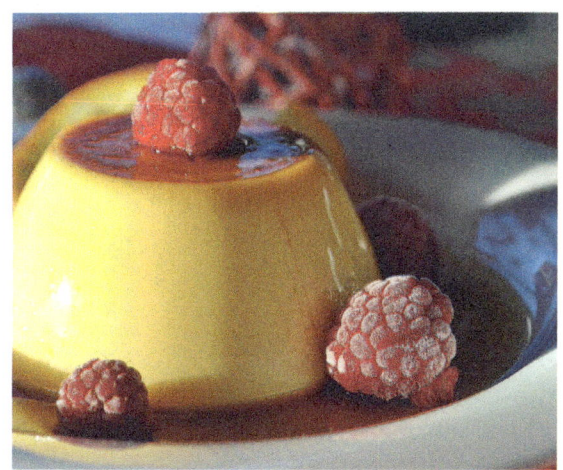

Ingredients:
- 1 cup sugar, divided
- 1/4 cup water
- 1 (14-ounce) can sweetened condensed milk
- 1 (12-ounce) can evaporated milk
- 6 eggs
- 1 teaspoon vanilla extract

Instructions:
1. Preheat oven to 350 degrees F and place 8 (6-ounce) ramekins into a large baking dish.
2. Add 1/2 cup sugar and water to a small saucepan then cook over medium heat, stirring constantly, until sugar has dissolved and mixture is bubbling. Cook for 1 minute then remove from heat and carefully pour into the bottom of one of the ramekins, tilting to coat the bottom evenly. Repeat with remaining ramekins.
3. In a large bowl, whisk together sweetened condensed milk, evaporated milk, eggs and vanilla until well combined.
4. Divide mixture evenly among the prepared ramekins then carefully pour enough hot water into the baking dish to come halfway up the sides of the ramekins.
5. Bake for 40-50 minutes or until custards are just set and slightly jiggly in the center. Remove from oven then allow to cool for 10 minutes.
6. Carefully remove ramekins from the water bath then refrigerate for at least 2 hours or overnight. Serve chilled.

Serving size: 1 ramekin
Calories: 330

SCONES

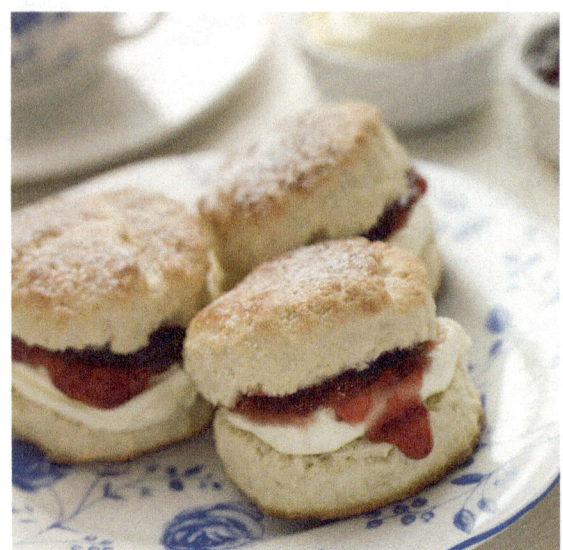

Ingredients:
- 2 cups gluten-free all-purpose flour
- 1 tablespoon baking powder
- 1/4 teaspoon salt
- 1/3 cup sugar
- 6 tablespoons cold butter, cut into small pieces
- 2/3 cup raisins
- 1 egg
- 1/2 cup milk

Instructions:
1. Preheat oven to 400 degrees F and line a baking sheet with parchment paper.
2. In a large bowl, whisk together flour, baking powder, salt and sugar. Cut in butter with a pastry blender or two knives until mixture resembles coarse crumbs. Stir in raisins.
3. In a small bowl, whisk together egg and milk then add to the flour mixture, stirring just until combined.
4. Drop dough by rounded tablespoons onto the prepared baking sheet then bake for 12-15 minutes or until scones are golden brown. Serve warm.

Serving size: 1 scone
Calories: 190

FROZEN FRUIT SORBET

Ingredients:
- 1 pound frozen fruit (strawberries, raspberries, blackberries, etc.)
- 1/2 cup sugar
- 1/2 cup water
- 1 tablespoon lemon juice

Instructions:
1. Add all ingredients to a blender or food processor then puree until smooth.
2. Pour mixture into an ice cream maker then freeze according to manufacturer's instructions. Serve immediately or store in the freezer for later.

Serving size: 1/2 cup
Calories: 130

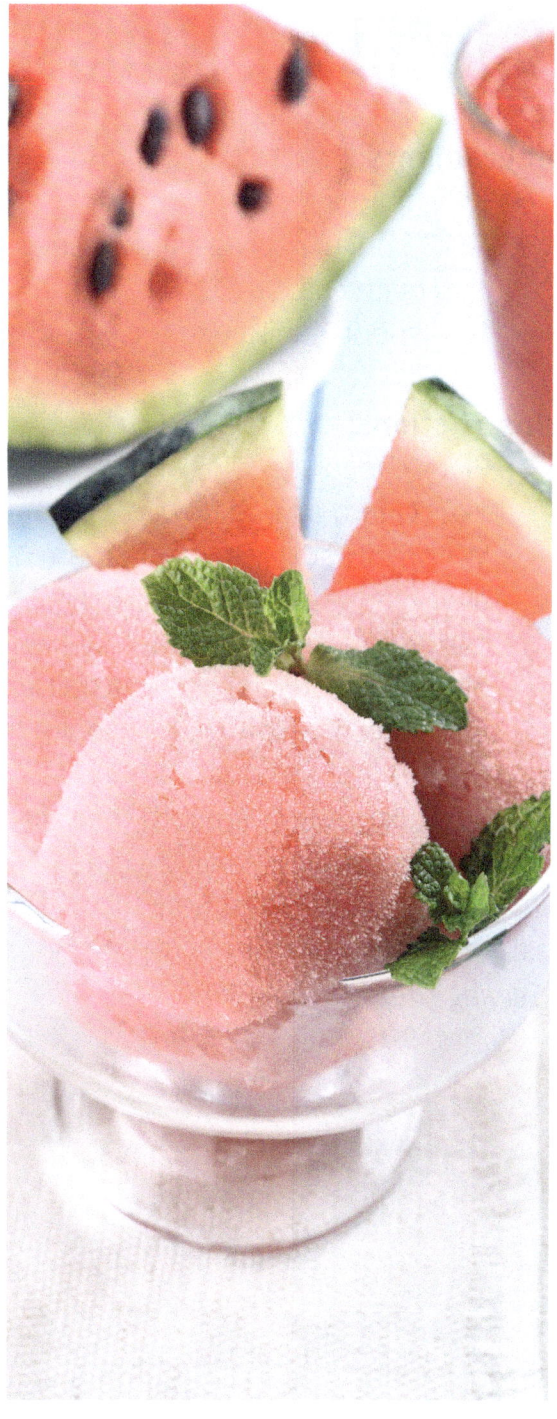

CHOCOLATE MOUSSE

Ingredients:
- 3/4 cup heavy cream
- 1 (12-ounce) package semi-sweet chocolate chips
- 1 teaspoon vanilla extract

Instructions:
1. Place chocolate chips and vanilla extract into a large bowl.
2. In a small saucepan, heat cream over medium heat until it just comes to a simmer. Pour hot cream over chocolate chips then let sit for 5 minutes to allow the chocolate to melt.
3. Stir mixture until smooth then refrigerate for at least 2 hours or overnight. Serve chilled.

Serving size: 1/2 cup
Calories: 310

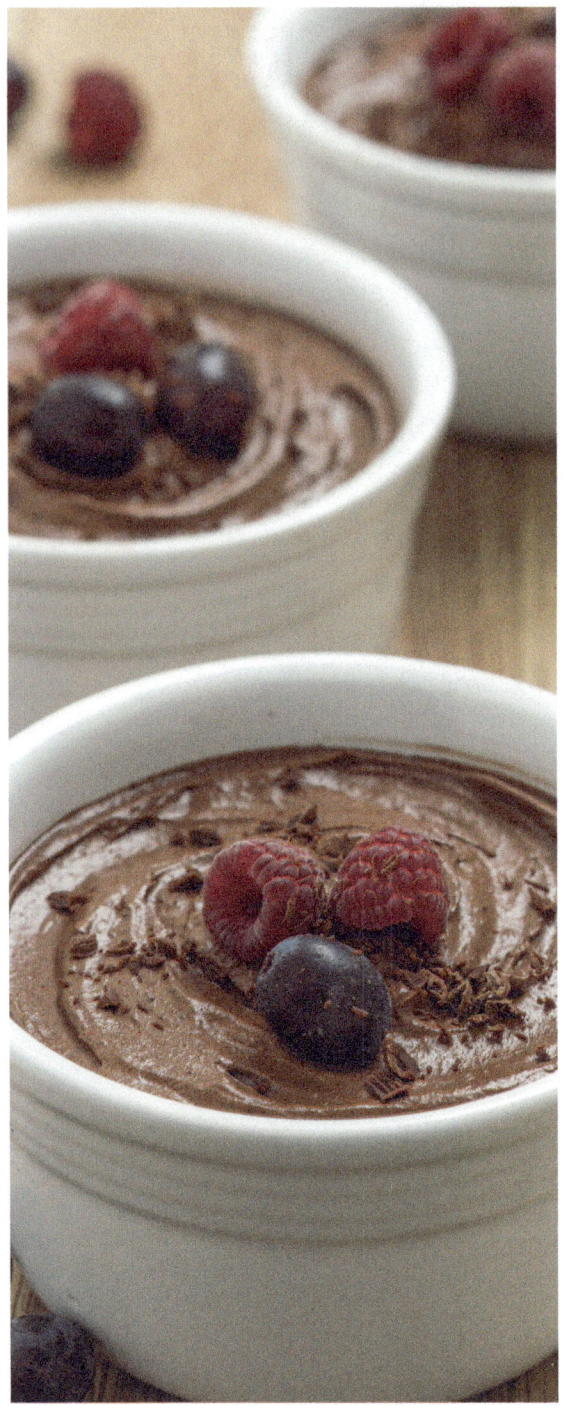

STRAWBERRY CHEESECAKE BITES

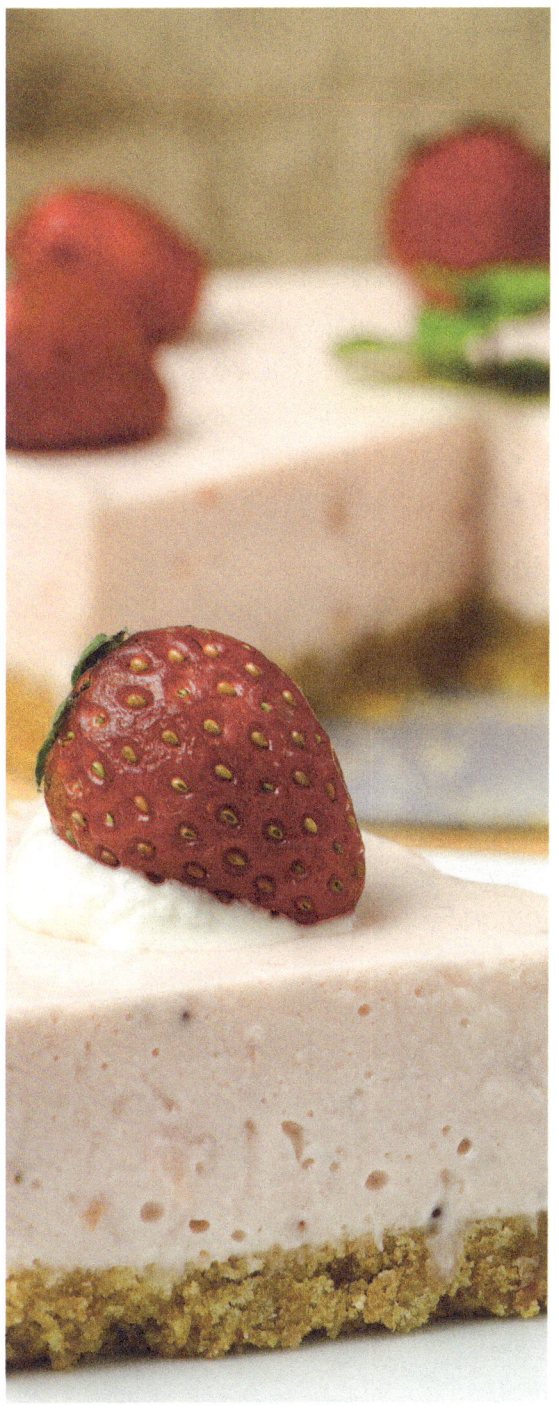

Ingredients:
- 1 (8-ounce) package cream cheese, softened
- 1/4 cup sugar
- 1 teaspoon vanilla extract
- 1 tablespoon gluten-free all-purpose flour
- 1 (10-ounce) package frozen strawberries, thawed and drained

Instructions:
1. Preheat oven to 350 degrees F and line a baking sheet with parchment paper.
2. In a medium bowl, beat together cream cheese, sugar, vanilla extract and flour until smooth. Gently stir in strawberries.
3. Drop mixture by rounded tablespoons onto the prepared baking sheet then bake for 15-20 minutes or until cheesecakes are set and golden brown. Serve warm or chilled.

Serving size: 1 cheesecake bite
Calories: 90

LEMON MERINGUE SMOOTHIE

Ingredients:
- 1 cup milk
- 1/2 cup plain yogurt
- 1/4 cup lemon juice
- 2 tablespoons honey
- 1 teaspoon vanilla extract
- 1/8 teaspoon salt

Instructions:
1. Add all ingredients to a blender or food processor then puree until smooth.
2. Pour mixture into glasses then serve immediately.

Serving size: 1 cup
Calories: 210

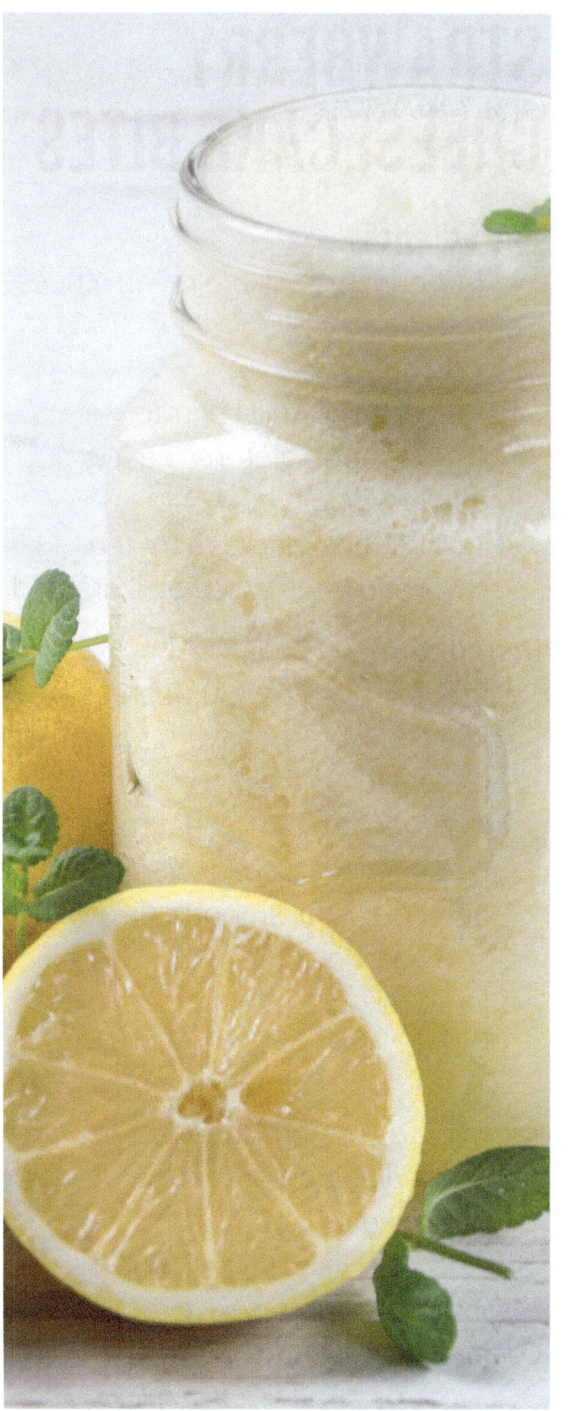

FROZEN YOGURT BITES

Ingredients:
- 1 cup plain yogurt
- 1/4 cup honey
- 1 teaspoon vanilla extract

Instructions:
1. Add all ingredients to a blender or food processor then puree until smooth.
2. Pour mixture into an ice cube tray then freeze for at least 6 hours or overnight. Serve frozen.

Serving size: 1 bite
Calories: 25

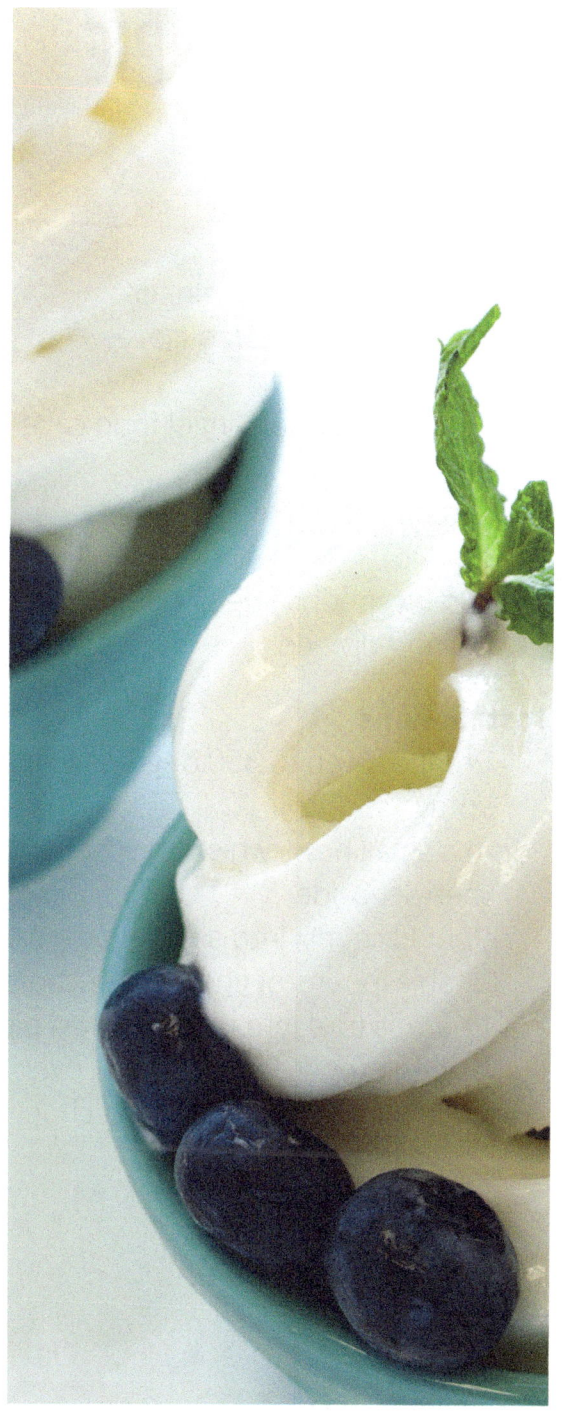

ANGEL PECAN PIE

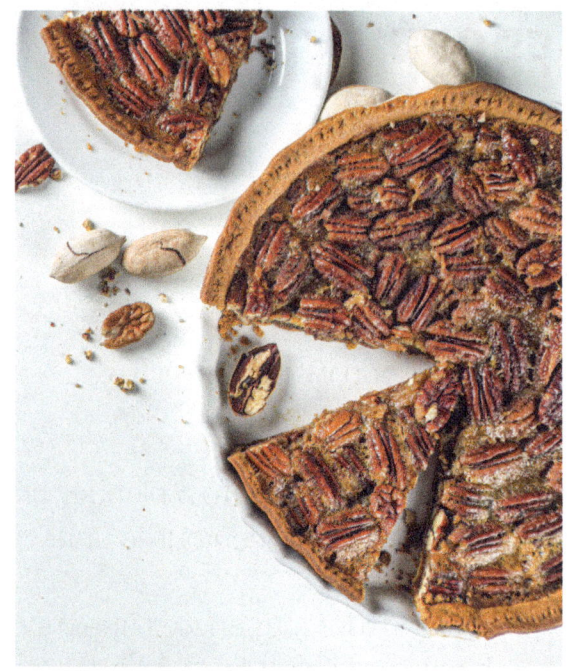

Ingredients:
- 1/2 cup sugar
- 1/4 cup cornstarch
- 1 teaspoon ground ginger
- 1/4 teaspoon ground cloves
- 1/8 teaspoon salt
- 1 (15-ounce) can angel food cake mix
- 2 tablespoons melted butter, divided
- 3 tablespoons finely chopped pecans, divided

Instructions:
1. Preheat oven to 350 degrees F and spray a 9-inch pie plate with cooking spray.
2. In a small bowl, whisk together sugar, cornstarch, ginger, cloves and salt then set aside.
3. Pour cake mix into a large bowl then add 1 tablespoon of melted butter and 2 tablespoons of chopped pecans, stirring until well combined.
4. Pour mixture into the prepared pie plate then bake for 25 minutes or until golden brown. Remove from oven then drizzle with remaining melted butter and sprinkle with remaining chopped pecans. Serve warm or chilled.

Serving size: 1 slice
Calories: 330

CHOCOLATE PUDDING

Ingredients:
- 1/2 cup sugar
- 1/3 cup cornstarch
- 1/4 cup unsweetened cocoa powder
- 1/8 teaspoon salt
- 2 cups milk, divided
- 1 teaspoon vanilla extract

Instructions:
1. In a medium saucepan, whisk together sugar, cornstarch, cocoa powder and salt then stir in 1 cup of milk.
2. Cook over medium heat, stirring constantly, until mixture comes to a boil then cook for 1 minute or until thickened. Remove from heat then stir in remaining milk and vanilla extract.
3. Pour pudding into individual bowls then serve immediately or refrigerate for later.

Serving size: 1/2 cup
Calories: 190

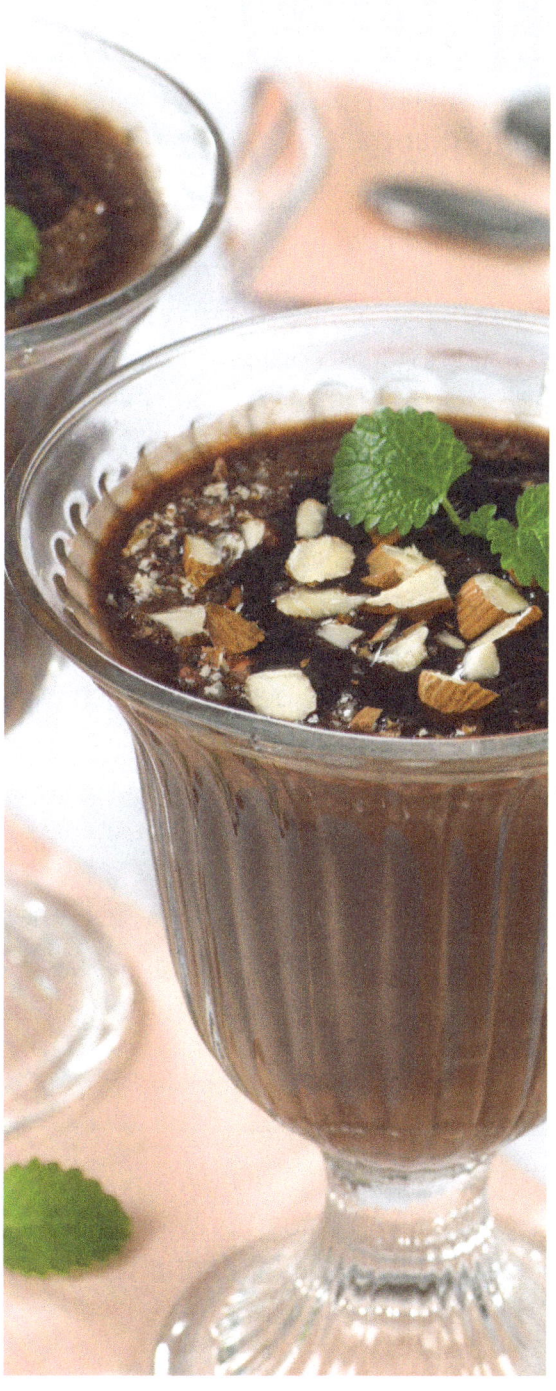

BLUEBERRY COBBLER

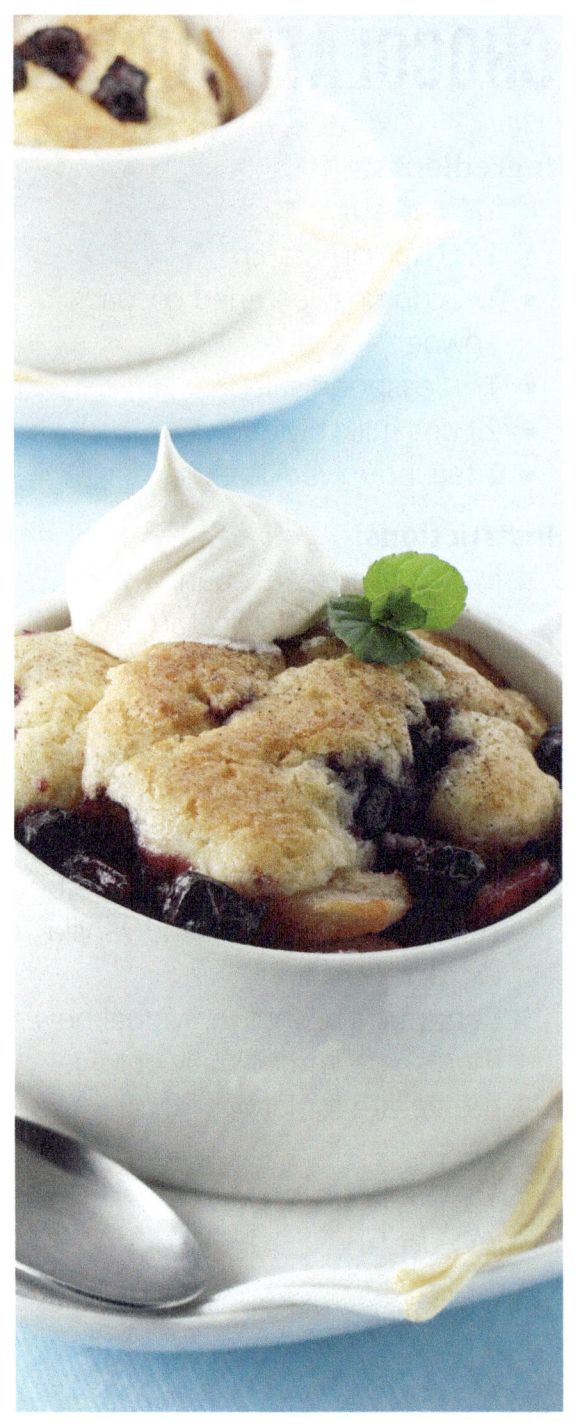

Ingredients:
- 1/2 cup sugar
- 1 tablespoon cornstarch
- 1/4 teaspoon ground cinnamon
- 1/8 teaspoon ground nutmeg
- 6 cups fresh or frozen blueberries, thawed
- 2 tablespoons lemon juice
- 1 recipe gluten-free biscuit dough (see below)

Instructions:
1. Preheat oven to 375 degrees F and spray a 9x13-inch baking dish with cooking spray.
2. In a small bowl, whisk together sugar, cornstarch, cinnamon and nutmeg then set aside.
3. In a large bowl, gently stir together blueberries and lemon juice then pour into the prepared baking dish. Sprinkle with sugar mixture then drop biscuit dough by rounded tablespoons over top.
4. Bake for 30-35 minutes or until cobbler is golden brown and bubbly. Serve warm or chilled.

Serving size: 1/2 cup
Calories: 270

PEACH CRISP

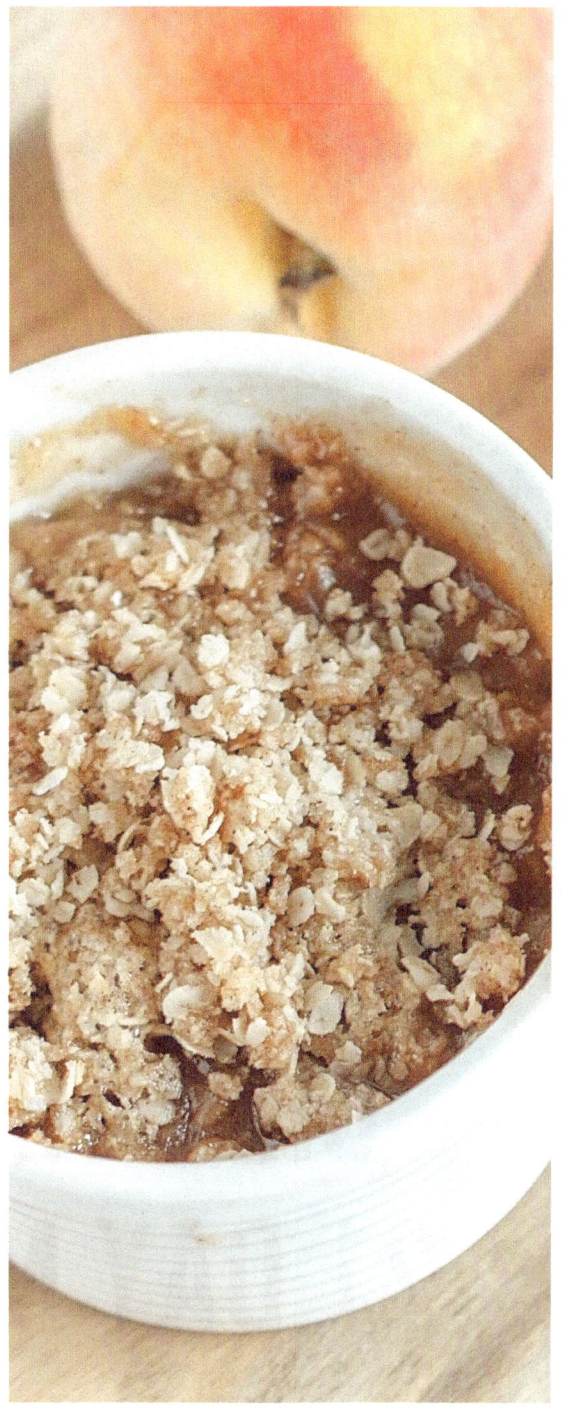

Ingredients:
- 1/2 cup sugar
- 1 tablespoon cornstarch
- 1 teaspoon ground cinnamon
- 1/4 teaspoon ground nutmeg
- 6 cups peeled and sliced fresh or frozen peaches, thawed
- 2 tablespoons lemon juice
- 1 recipe gluten-free crisp topping (see below)

Instructions:
1. Preheat oven to 375 degrees F and spray a 9x13-inch baking dish with cooking spray.
2. In a small bowl, whisk together sugar, cornstarch, cinnamon and nutmeg then set aside.
3. In a large bowl, gently stir together peaches and lemon juice then pour into the prepared baking dish. Sprinkle with sugar mixture then top with crisp topping.
4. Bake for 30-35 minutes or until crisp is golden brown and bubbly. Serve warm or chilled.

Serving size: 1/2 cup
Calories: 320

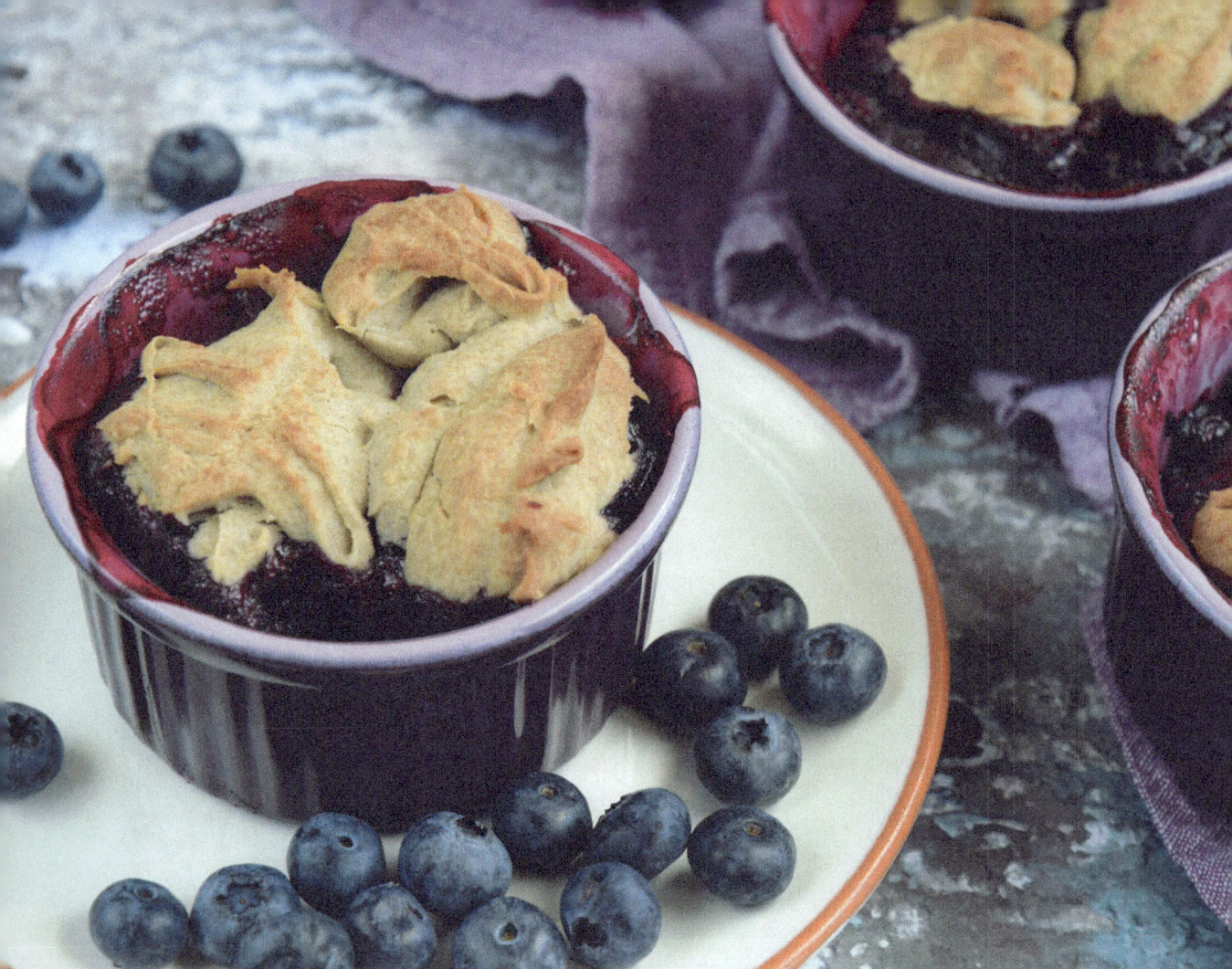

CHAPTER SEVEN: 21 DAY MEAL PLAN

21-DAY MEAL PLAN

Day 1:
Snack: Fruit and Nut Bars ..page 3
Breakfast: Banana Oatmeal ..page 33
Lunch: Tomato Basil Soup ..page 59
Dinner: Beef Stir Fry with Broccoli and Brown Rice ..page 85
Dessert: Sugar Cookies ..page 116

Day 2:
Snack: Banana Sushi ..page 10
Breakfast: Quinoa Breakfast Bowl ..page 47
Lunch: Curried Lentil Soup ..page 58
Dinner: Turkey Chili ..page 97
Dessert: Lemon Meringue Smoothie ..page 130

Day 3:
Snack: Apple Nachos ..page 11
Breakfast: Breakfast Tacos ..page 30
Lunch: Spicy Thai Peanut Noodles ..page 55
Dinner: Shepherd's Pie ..page 99
Dessert: Brownies ..page 112

Day 4:
Snack: Edamame ..page 17
Breakfast: Banana Pancakes ..page 46
Lunch: Quinoa Pilaf ..page 69
Dinner: Baked Ham with Sweet Potato Casserole and Green Beans ..page 98
Dessert: Oreo Cheesecake Bites ..page 117

Day 5:
Snack: Watermelon with Mint ..page 25
Breakfast: Blueberry Almond Pancakes ..page 29
Lunch: White Bean Chicken Chili ..page 60
Dinner: Meatloaf with Mashed Potatoes and Carrots ..page 102
Dessert: Tiramisu ..page 124

Day 6:
Snack: Orange with Almond Butter ..page 21
Breakfast: Omelet with Vegetables ..page 43
Lunch: Thai Chicken Wraps ..page 64
Dinner: Spaghetti Squash with Turkey Meat Sauce ..page 92
Dessert: Peach Cobbler ..page 120

Day 7:
Snack: Cauliflower Popcorn ..page 16
Breakfast: Green Smoothie ..page 39
Lunch: Eggplant Parmesan ..page 67
Dinner: Salmon Cakes with Roasted Vegetables ..page 100
Dessert: Angel Pecan Pie ..page 132

Day 8:
Snack: Veggie Chips ..page 26
Breakfast: Peach and Arugula Salad ..page 32
Lunch: Turkey and Apple Sandwich on Gluten-Free Bread ..page 65
Dinner: Chicken Pot Pie ..page 108
Dessert: Flan ..page 125

Day 9:
Snack: Celery Sticks with Peanut Butter ..page 15
Breakfast: Quiche ..page 41
Lunch: Spicy Black Bean Soup ..page 57
Dinner: Turkey Burger with Sweet Potato Fries ..page 86
Dessert: Strawberry Shortcake ..page 118

Day 10:
Snack: Roasted Chickpeas ..page 2
Breakfast: Scrambled Eggs with Spinach and Cheese ..page 44
Lunch: Sautéed Shrimp with Zucchini Noodles and Pesto ..page 63
Dinner: Chicken and Broccoli Stir Fry ..page 80
Dessert: Blueberry Crisp ..page 111

Day 11:
Snack: Cantaloupe with Cottage Cheese ..page 20
Breakfast: Grilled Cheese Sandwich ..page 40
Lunch: Meat and Vegetable Rollups ..page 72
Dinner: One Pot BBQ Chicken and Quinoa ..page 83
Dessert: Chocolate Mousse ..page 129

Day 12:
Snack: Parmesan Garlic Kale Chips ..page 7
Breakfast: Cinnamon Roll Baked Oatmeal ..page 31
Lunch: Pink Salmon Salad with Vegetables ..page 76
Dinner: Salmon with Quinoa and Roasted Vegetables ..page 94
Dessert: Chocolate Chip Cookies ..page 113

Day 13:
Snack: Cucumber Bites ..page 12
Breakfast: Egg Breakfast Sandwich ..page 37
Lunch: Spicy Black Bean Burger with Avocado Mayo and Roasted Sweet Potato Wedges ..page 61
Dinner: Crockpot Honey Garlic Chicken ..page 82
Dessert: Peanut Butter Cookies ..page 115

Day 14:
Snack: Cucumber Avocado Tea Sandwiches ..page 4
Breakfast: Sausage and Egg Breakfast Burrito ..page 45
Lunch: Quinoa Salad with Roasted Vegetables ..page 62
Dinner: Grilled Chicken with Roasted Vegetables ..page 81
Dessert: Scones ..page 126

Day 15:
Snack: Trail Mix ..page 9
Breakfast: Banana Bread Overnight Oats ..page 28
Lunch: Spaghetti Squash with Tomato Sauce ..page 66
Dinner: Lentil Soup ..page 91
Dessert: Peach Crisp ..page 135

Day 16:
Snack: Carrot Sticks with Hummus ..page 14
Breakfast: Avocado Toast ..page 50
Lunch: Greek Yogurt Chicken Salad ..page 56
Dinner: Roasted Pork Loin with Sweet Potatoes and Apples ..page 105
Dessert: Chocolate Chip Banana Bread ..page 110

Day 17:
Snack: Cherry Tomatoes with Basil ..page 13
Breakfast: Blueberry Muffins ..page 34
Lunch: Turkey Wrap ..page 68
Dinner: Quinoa Salad with Grilled Chicken ..page 89
Dessert: Vanilla Pudding ..page 122

Day 18:
Snack: Sweet Potato Chips ..page 6
Breakfast: Cinnamon Rolls ..page 36
Lunch: Chickpea Salad ..page 70
Dinner: Roasted Chicken with Roasted Vegetables ..page 93
Dessert: Chocolate Covered Strawberries ..page 119

Day 19:
Snack: Fruit Kabobs ..page 18
Breakfast: Chocolate Chip Pancakes ..page 35
Lunch: Tomato Basil Chicken ..page 78
Dinner: Beef Stew with Potatoes and Carrots ..page 96
Dessert: Frozen Yogurt Bites ..page 131

Day 20:
Snack: Pineapple with Coconut Milk ..page 23
Breakfast: Banana Pancakes ..page 46
Lunch: Garlic Mashed Potatoes ..page 71
Dinner: Beef Stroganoff ..page 101
Dessert: Crème Brulee ..page 123

Day 21:
Snack: Strawberry with Balsamic Vinegar ..page 24
Breakfast: Quinoa Breakfast Bowl ..page 47
Lunch: Quinoa Salad with Cranberries and Feta ..page 74
Dinner: Roasted Turkey Breast with Stuffing and Green Beans ..page 103
Dessert: Blueberry Cobbler ..page 134

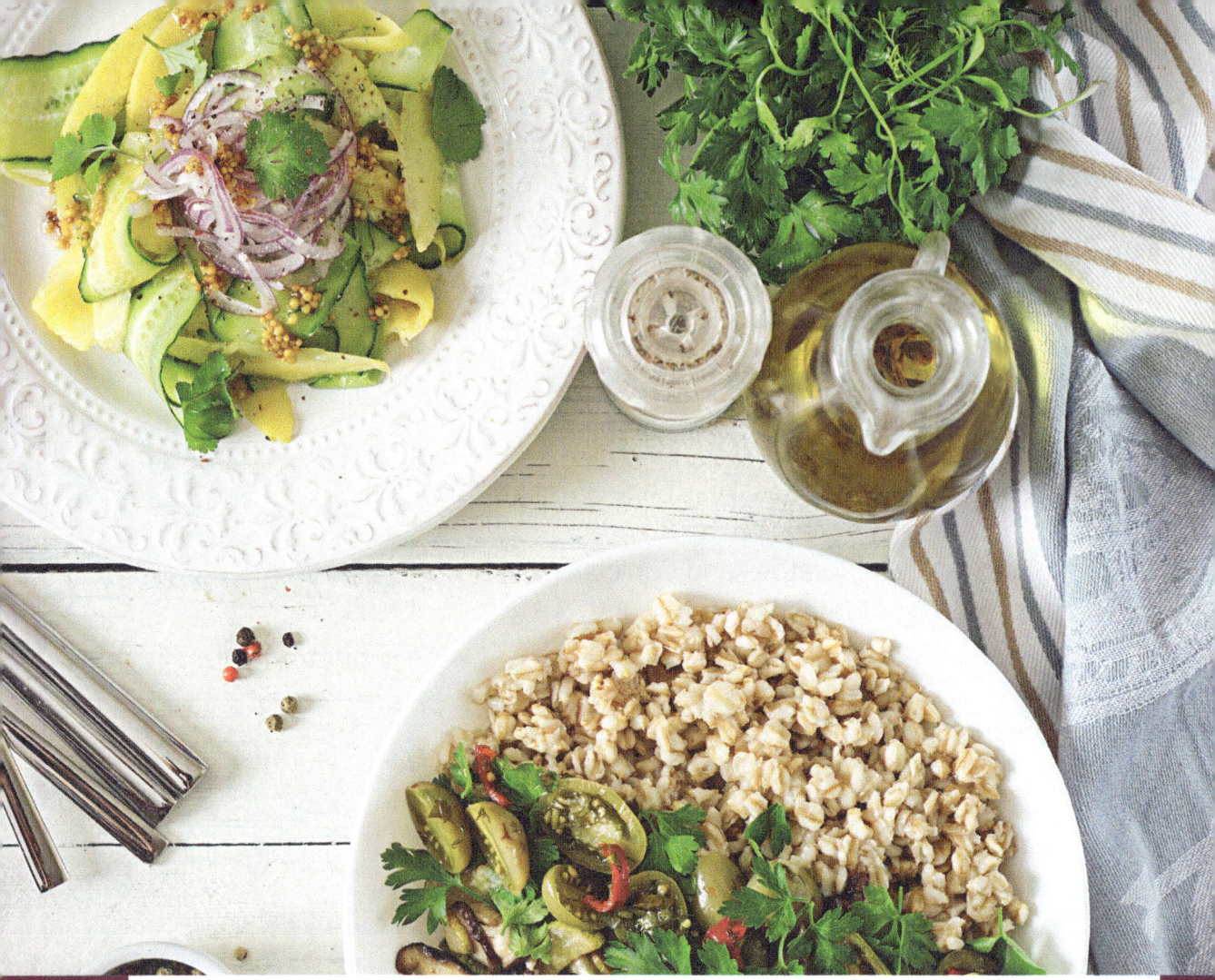

ABOUT THE AUTHOR

RAPID HEALING MADE EASY

I suffered for nearly a decade and a half with no answers and was resigned to the reality that I would never get better, and it was only a matter of time before the disease took the rest of my life.

Until I discovered Acemannan.

I first learned about this rare aloe vera molecule during a tax strategy call for my book publishing business. After we saved me an additional $20,000 for my previous two years of tax returns, our discussion shifted to kingdom building and health.

I learned my tax strategist had also suffered from serious health problems for a decade and a half before she found full recovery and healing. Naturally, I dug deeper to find out more about what she did.

It was therapeutic supplements from a company called Manna- Relief who provided organic, immune boosting nutrition to malnourished children all around the world. They were saving kids' lives who were forgotten, and left to die at orphanages with no answers to why they too were sick and dying.

It turned out they had a similar problem as me, manifested in a different form. We both had disrupted and damaged immune systems and gut microbiomes. Due to this our bodies were unable to heal itself properly and were more easily subject to chronic disease, infection, and chronic inflammation.

While they didn't have enough nutrition, my body was killing itself unintentionally because of rampant bacterial infections raging in my colon. Yet, the solution was the same—restore the gut and activate the immune system. It sounded like science fiction to me as she explained the thera- peutics and incredible results people were experiencing with it.

Things like:

- Cancers
- Tumors
- Cystic fibrosis
- Fibromyalgia
- AIDs
- IBD
- IBS (IBS-D, IBS-C)
- Ulcerative colitis
- Pancolitis
- Diverticulitis
- Celiac disease
- Crohn's disease
- Alzheimer's
- Dementia
- Sickle cell anemia
- Fungal infections
- Bacterial infections
- Chronic infections
- Viruses
- Coronavirus (Covid-19)
- Autoimmune diseases
- Chronic fatigue syndrome
- Arthritis
- Migraines
- Allergies
- Eczema
- Dwarfism
- Chronic inflammation
- Hormonal disorders
- Lymphatic disorders
- And many more

To say I was skeptical was an understatement. Yet, I was open- minded enough to listen and ask questions for the off chance it might work for me too. One young boy had a rare and inoperable eye tumor when his family learned about Acemannan. They put him on these non-toxic, non-biological altering therapeutics and within six months his tumor was completely gone.

When I saw a before and after picture of this young boy it was as though the tumor had never been there. I figured it had been years for that result and why I asked them how long it had been for the boy. Six months.

That's how long it took for his body to completely wipe out that tumor, and restore his life and face. And all he did differently was take these therapeutics that had the strongest anti fungal, antiviral, anti-inflammatory, and immune boosting nutrients from the aloe vera plant, New Zealand pine park, New Zealand Manuka flow- ering plant, and beets.

At this point my "this is too good to be true" radar was off the charts. How could natural and holistic therapeutics be enabling people's bodies to heal from serious illnesses and diseases? I thought these were all incurable and that only vaccines and medications could mitigate, cure, or heal disease.

But then I got to the point of no return. I could yield to my skepticism and belief that nothing would work, or I could give it a try. I literally said out loud on my tax strategy call, "I'll try it. What do I have to lose?"

I ordered one bottle and haven't had any issues with ulcer- ative colitis, or any of my symptoms and health problems, since.

What you've found in this book is information about ulcerative colitis, what it is, its symptoms, and what helps during flare ups. I also included common foods to avoid during a flare up, what foods to eat that won't irritate your colon too much while still providing you with nutrients, meal plans, recipes, and grocery lists to make your healing journey as painless and simple as possible.

I know when I was on my journey to recovery it was terrifying and filled with confusion as I had no idea what to do, what to eat or not eat, and how to actually find true and lasting healing—if it existed.

The good news is it does.

Use this cookbook as your roadmap to managing your flare ups with more peace of mind, and ultimately, find total restoration like I did.

If you'd like to learn more about the therapeutics I took (and still do) that completely healed my body within two weeks, you can click the link to learn more.

https://operationlove.myalovea.com

If you're at a place like I was (and hopefully you'll never get there) where you're able to say, "What do I have to lose? Let me try them like Matthew did and see what they do for me."

Then you should seriously consider checking them out for your-self to learn more at the very minimum. I'm not saying it'll heal or cure you of disease as the FDA says it's illegal to claim anything but vaccines and medications cure, mitigate, or heal disease—even if they do.

All I'm saying is, "Why not give it a try and find out for yourself?" Ulcerative colitis is a lonely and dark road, but now you don't have to stay in the darkness any longer. I hope this book helps you with meal prep, foods, healing, and gaining your life back.

The world needs you in it, and we need you at your top self to reach your full potential and impact the world with your presence. My hope for you is that you experience recovery and healing like I did, and many others before me. You don't have to suffer with this disease by yourself or without answers. There are solutions out there that are working for people like you and me.

Pick one and find your healing. If you're curious what I took, here's the list (and still take every day):
Immun, Limitless, Daily, Balance, Cell-a-brate

You can learn more about these and all of Alovea's products at: https://operationlove.myalovea.com.myalovea.com.

If you end up getting some, use the referral code *OPERATIONLOVE* to get 15% off your orders.

If you'd like to donate to help fund the mission to provide nutri-tion to malnourished kids around the world, then check out Manna-Relief at https://www.mannarelief.org/.

OPERATION LOVE

If you'd like to join a community of likeminded people who are going through the same thing you are, found healing, or to experi- ence support while you go through it, then come join us at **Operation Love.**

We'd love to have you join us, and let us support you, encourage you, and help you on your healing journey too. We have an open Facebook group for people to come together with one mission: find healing from disease.

And if you've experienced healing yourself, we'd love to hear your story. Come share it with us! You never know when your words and story might change some- one's life and give them that extra push to keep going and not give up. Find us on Facebook at:

Operation Love — Providing Educational Resources For Healing Of Disease

ABOUT MATTHEW THRUSH

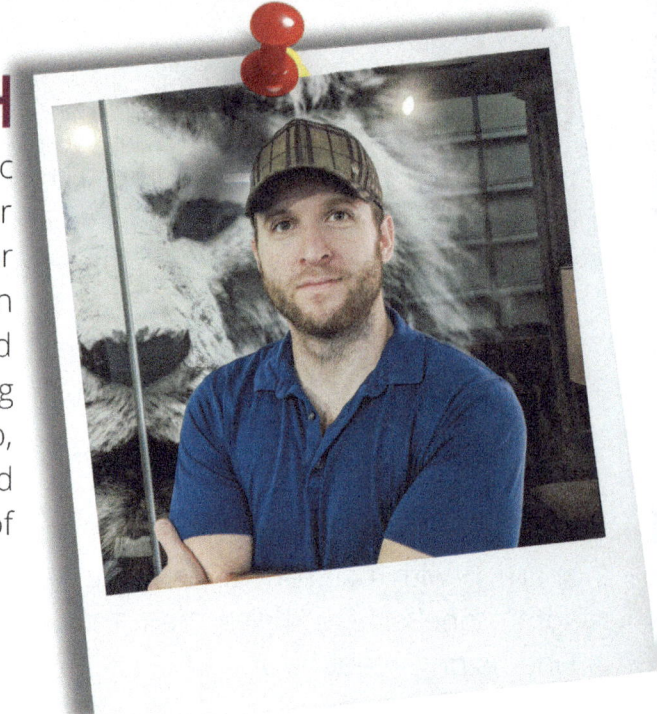

Matthew suffered from chronic inflammatory bowel disease (IBD) for over a decade with no answers or improvement. His health issues began as extreme vertigo, nausea, and vomiting on a daily basis after being given vaccines during Naval Boot Camp, and worsened as the years progressed through constant prescription of antibiotics and NSAIDs.

Soon, these evolved into daily migraines, severe allergies, chronic pain, insomnia, anxiety, and abdominal complications (blood, diar- rhea, fecal incontinence, and constant bathroom visits) that resulted in him being bed- and toilet-ridden for three years at its peak.

His marriage suffered. His relationship with his friends, family, and two sons was nonexistent. And he could not get promoted at his job due to his constant absence from work for doctor appointments, or requiring to rush home to shower and change because he had another "accident".

He tried several diets and protocols from various gastrointestinal specialists with minor relief—oftentimes, with no improvement. When he found MannaRelief in Dallas, TX, everything changed within two weeks.

He tried their therapeutic supplements and noticed radical improve- ments within four days—his bathroom visits every 15 minutes with bloody stools stopped. After about two weeks of taking their prod- uct, infused with Acemannan, all of his health complications had vanished as though he had never had them.

The only lingering demon he still needed to crush was renewing his mind that he was actually healed and no longer sick, which meant training his thoughts that he could re-engage with the world and not worry about panic attacks crippling him anytime he was more than ten minutes from a bathroom.

His mission is to eradicate diseases caused by chronic inflammation and restore hope to people so they can get their lives back like he did.

He shares what he has learned through his years of pursuit for answers, the science and evidence he found for total gut restoration, and ultimately, sharing his story of what healed his body completely so others can experience the same outcome.

You can learn more about Matthew's journey and the life-changing therapeutics he takes and now shares with everyone at

https://www.operationlove.com/myalovea.com.

ALSO BY MATTHEW THRUSH

Whole Body Healing
- The Ulcerative Colitis Diet Cookbook
- The Irritable Bowel Syndrome Diet Cookbook
- The Bloating, Gas, & Abdominal Discomfort Diet Cookbook
- The Crohn's Disease Diet Cookbook
- The Diverticulitis Diet Cookbook
- The Diabetes Diet Cookbook
- The Migraines Diet Cookbook
- The Celiac Disease Diet Cookbook
- The Seasonal Allergies Diet Cookbook
- The Sinusitis Diet Cookbook
- The Chronic Fatigue Diet Cookbook
- The Weight Loss Diet Cookbook
- The Chronic Pain Diet Cookbook
- The Arthritis, Joint, Neck, & Back Pain Diet Cookbook
- The Youthful Energy Diet Cookbook
- The Anti-Aging Diet Cookbook
- The Gut Health & Immunity Diet Cookbook
- The Viruses, Bacterial Infections, Colds, & Flus Diet Cookbook
- The Body Detox Diet Cookbook

Total Gut Makeover
- Total Gut Makeover: Ulcerative Colitis
- Total Gut Makeover: IBS
- Total Gut Makeover: Crohn's Disease
- Total Gut Makeover: Diabetes
- Total Gut Makeover: Cystic Fibrosis
- Total Gut Makeover: Diverticulitis
- Total Gut Makeover: Gut Health & Immunity
- Total Gut Makeover: Irritable Bowel Disease (IBD)
- Total Gut Makeover: Small Intestinal Bacterial Overgrowth (SIBO)
- Total Gut Makeover: Sinusitis
- Total Gut Makeover: Migraines
- Total Gut Makeover: Celiac Disease
- Total Gut Makeover: Diabetes
- Total Gut Makeover: Chronic Fatigue Syndrome

ALSO BY MATTHEW THRUSH

Total Body Rejuvenation
- The Complete Anti-Inflammatory Cookbook For Ulcerative Colitis:
- The Complete Anti-Inflammatory Cookbook For Diabetes
- The Complete Anti-Inflammatory Cookbook For Crohn's Disease
- The Complete Anti-Inflammatory Cookbook For Irritable Bowel Disease
- The Complete Anti-Inflammatory Cookbook For Bloating, Gas, & Abdominal Discomfort
- The Complete Anti-Inflammatory Cookbook For Seasonal Allergies
- The Complete Anti-Inflammatory Cookbook For Sinusitis
- The Complete Anti-Inflammatory Cookbook For Migraines
- The Complete Anti-Inflammatory Cookbook For Chronic Fatigue
- The Complete Anti-Inflammatory Cookbook For Weight Loss
- The Complete Anti-Inflammatory Cookbook For Chronic Pain
- The Complete Anti-Inflammatory Cookbook For Arthritis, Joint, Neck, & Back Pain
- The Complete Anti-Inflammatory Cookbook For Youthful Energy
- The Complete Anti-Inflammatory Cookbook For Anti-Aging
- The Complete Anti-Inflammatory Cookbook For Gut Health & Immunity
- The Complete Anti-Inflammatory Cookbook For Viruses, Bacterial Infections, Colds, & Flus
- The Complete Anti-Inflammatory Cookbook For Detoxing The Body

INDEX

A
- Angel Pecan Pie .. 132
- Apple Nachos .. 11
- Avocado Toast .. 50

B
- Baked Ham With Sweet Potato Casserole and Green Beans .. 97
- Banana Bread Overnight Oats .. 28
- Banana Oatmeal .. 33
- Banana Pancakes .. 46
- Banana Sushi .. 10
- Beef Stew .. 107
- Beef Stew with Potatoes and Carrots .. 95
- Beef Stir Fry with Broccoli and Brown Rice .. 85
- Beef Stroganoff .. 101
- Blueberry Almond Pancakes .. 29
- Blueberry Cobbler .. 134
- Blueberry Crisp .. 110
- Blueberry Muffins .. 34
- Breakfast Smoothie .. 48
- Breakfast Tacos .. 30
- Brownies .. 112

C
- Cantaloupe with Cottage Cheese .. 20
- Carrot Sticks with Hummus .. 14
- Cauliflower Popcorn .. 16
- Celery Sticks with Peanut Butter .. 15
- Cherry Tomatoes with Basil .. 13
- Chicken and Broccoli Stir Fry .. 80
- Chicken Curry with Coconut Milk and Rice .. 94
- Chicken Pot Pie .. 108
- Chickpea Salad .. 70
- Chocolate Chip Banana Bread .. 110
- Chocolate Chip Cookies .. 113
- Chocolate Chip Pancakes .. 35
- Chocolate Covered Strawberries .. 119
- Chocolate Hummus .. 5
- Chocolate Mousse .. 128
- Chocolate Pudding .. 133
- Cinnamon Roll Baked Oatmeal .. 31
- Cinnamon Rolls .. 36
- Crème Brulee .. 123
- Crockpot Honey Garlic Chicken .. 82
- Cucumber Avocado Tea Sandwiches .. 4
- Cucumber Bites .. 12
- Curried Lentil Soup .. 58

E
- Edamame .. 17
- Egg Breakfast Sandwich .. 37
- Eggplant Parmesan .. 67

F
- Flan .. 125
- Frozen Fruit Sorbet .. 127
- Frozen Yogurt Bites .. 131
- Fruit and Nut Bars .. 3
- Fruit Kabobs .. 18
- Fruit Salad .. 38

INDEX

G
- Garden Veggie Soup .. 73
- Garlic Mashed Potatoes .. 71
- Grapefruit with Honey .. 19
- Greek Yogurt Chicken Salad .. 56
- Greek Yogurt with Fruit and Honey .. 49
- Green Smoothie .. 39
- Grilled Cheese Sandwich .. 40
- Grilled Chicken with Roasted Vegetables .. 81

L
- Lemon Meringue Smoothie .. 130
- Lentil Soup .. 90

M
- Meat and Vegetable Rollups .. 72
- Meatloaf with Mashed Potatoes and Carrots .. 102

O
- Oatmeal Chocolate Chip Cookies .. 114
- Omelet with Vegetables .. 43
- One Pot BBQ Chicken and Quinoa .. 83
- Orange with Almond Butter .. 21
- Oreo Cheesecake Bites .. 117

P
- Parmesan Garlic Kale Chips .. 7
- Peach and Arugula Salad .. 32
- Peach Cobbler .. 120
- Peach Crisp .. 135
- Peach with Yogurt .. 22
- Peanut Butter Cookies .. 115
- Pineapple with Coconut Milk .. 23
- Pink Salmon Salad with Vegetables .. 76
- Potato Soup with Bacon, Cheese, and Scallions .. 75

Q
- Quiche .. 41
- Quinoa Breakfast Bowl .. 47
- Quinoa Pilaf .. 69
- Quinoa Salad with Cranberries and Feta .. 74
- Quinoa Salad with Grilled Chicken .. 88
- Quinoa Salad with Roasted Vegetables .. 62
- Quinoa Veggie Bowl .. 54

R
- Roasted Chicken with Roasted Vegetables .. 92
- Roasted Chickpeas .. 2
- Roasted Pork Loin with Sweet Potatoes and Apples .. 105
- Roasted Turkey Breast with Stuffing and Green Beans .. 103

S
- Salmon Cakes with Roasted Vegetables .. 100
- Salmon with Quinoa and Roasted Vegetables .. 93
- Salmon with Roasted Brussels Sprouts .. 84
- Sausage and Egg Breakfast Burrito .. 45

INDEX

- Sautéed Shrimp with Zucchini Noodles and Pesto .. 63
- Scones .. 126
- Scrambled Eggs with Spinach and Cheese .. 44
- Shepherd's Pie .. 99
- Smoked Salmon Bagel .. 51
- Spaghetti Squash with Tomato Sauce .. 66
- Spaghetti Squash with Turkey Meat Sauce .. 91
- Spicy Black Bean Burger with Avocado Mayo and Roasted Sweet Potato Wedges .. 57
- Spicy Black Bean Soup .. 8
- Spicy Roasted Edamame .. 77
- Spicy Sausage and Kale Soup .. 55
- Spicy Thai Peanut Noodles .. 129
- Strawberry Cheesecake Bites ..
- Strawberry Shortcake .. 118
- Strawberry with Balsamic Vinegar .. 24
- Sugar Cookies .. 116
- Sweet Potato Chips .. 6

T
- Thai Chicken Wraps .. 64
- Tiramisu .. 124
- Tomato Basil Chicken .. 78
- Tomato Basil Soup .. 59
- Tomato Soup .. 42
- Trail Mix .. 9
- Turkey and Apple Sandwich on Gluten-Free Bread .. 65
- Turkey Burger with Sweet Potato Fries .. 86
- Turkey Chili .. 96
- Turkey Wrap .. 68

V
- Vanilla Pudding .. 122
- Vegetable Lasagna .. 106
- Veggie Chips .. 26

W
- Watermelon with Mint .. 25
- White Bean Chicken Chili .. 60

Y
- Yogurt Parfait .. 52

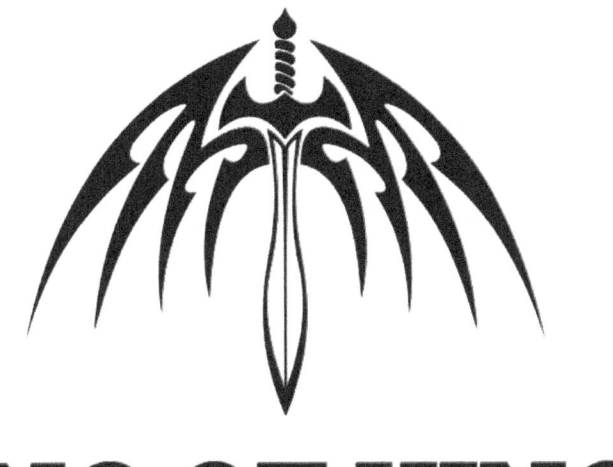

KING OF KINGS

Copyright © 2022 Matthew Thrush

All rights reserved. No part of this guide may be reproduced in any form without permission in writing from the publisher except in the case of brief quotations embodied in critical articles or reviews.

Made in the USA
Coppell, TX
18 June 2023